To Nikola and Leon, who I love dearly.

I dedicate this book to my niece Nicola and nephew Leon and I trust they will understand how sorry I am, not to have seen them as often as I would have wished.

CONTENTS

Magic Roundabout

1) Take the Exit & I will Survive this Family 1

2) Crazy Emotions & Enough is Enough 27

3) Carousel & Losing my Mind 47

4) Fat and Fatter, Slim and Slimmer & Am I going to Die? 72

5) Slow is Steady, Steady is Fast & Firing Field 89

6) Vegans, Empaths and Buddha & All that you have is your Soul .108

7) How We Do It & Beautiful Dreamer 124

8) Fast Car & My Red Pill Therapy 142

9) Food Everywhere 169

10) That Place called the Gym & The Face of Change 248

References

Why this book?

Well, there are a few reasons. This book is a thank you to some amazing souls that helped me get back on my feet after a very stressful time.

I was not so lucky with my biological family, and some strangers in life became my family. They were sent from heaven, and I realize that not everyone is this lucky.

I had some roundabouts in my life that led me to exhaustion. I was at my lowest, and I did not believe I could fix things. I was lucky, and met some amazing people, and those people then led me to key books. I ended up reading over twenty psychology and self-help books, and I was very emotional as I realised that if someone had told me much of this earlier, I would have saved myself lots of pain. Many people just like me have no idea why they have roundabouts in their life, and without the relevant knowledge, it's pretty hard.

When I worked as a personal trainer, I sometimes felt more like a psychologist as my clients would off-load and share their personal problems with me. I realised that many of us need more help and knowledge, but without someone who is either qualified or has been through it, it's nearly impossible to get the help we need.

Many amazing people are struggling, but literally feel stuck as they don't know how to fix things. As many people offloaded, I realized how much people bottle up without self-help, and rather kept everything inside. It felt like it was slowly eating their and my soul away.

In each chapter, I am putting small hints, and at the end, I am explaining some terms that might be beneficial for you guys that are going through difficult times; maybe you don't know where to look or what is actually going on, and why you feel the way you do.

There are some YouTube videos from people that know what they are talking about and some great books that helped me massively to understand. I have found in the books explanations for everything that was putting question marks into my head and more. The knowledge is fascinating. This book is here to make you smile, but mainly I hope it's going to point you towards what you need to sort out, the problems that might be breaking you. I also want you guys to understand that you can have the body you desire no matter what roundabouts with diets you have. Your body is a souls' house. We should all look after it.

Thank you to all the people that were honest, truthful, and never judged. They always saw more good than bad in others and me. To people that helped without expecting anything back, and to people that knew the struggles, and they did not let others suffer when they had the ability to help. To those who choose to do the right thing at a spiritual level, and to people that are not blinded by the opinion of others.

A massive thank you to my darling sister Rashmi, who I have been very lucky to have in my life. To David Wintle, who I worked for. He affected my life the most of all people I have met. Life would be so poor without the goodness in people.

Sometimes people are the best thing that can happen to us, and sometimes the worst one.

Magic Roundabouts

Do you live in England? I do. And one thing I was amazed by when I moved to this country were roundabouts. They were everywhere. Soon I learnt that if I didn't know where I was or what to do, I could just go around and around until I felt dizzy. I loved it. Like on a carousel!

When I got to Swindon, where my close friend lived, and the first time I've seen the magic roundabout, I thought this looks just like my life at the moment! Chaos, but somehow an organized one.

Later on, I even thought to myself that English people never get to the point, but they politely use the roundabout everywhere, thank goodness not the magic one as we would be all lost. I still haven't worked out if it's a good thing or a bad thing. But I got used to it.

After I qualified as a personal trainer and started working in the fitness industry, I realized that most people use the gym as a roundabout without getting to the destination. But what amazed me more was the fact that most people never came to me and asked me the question ... "I've been to the gym nearly every day.

I've worked really hard for the last three years, and not much has changed! Should I not look like a supermodel or Arnie by now? Yes, you should! In fact, you were supposed to look like that last year. What have you been doing?

But I am not going to bore you here with all this stuff. After asking a few people this question, as I was curious myself, the answer I received back amazed me even more. They believed that this is the best they can look, as they worked really hard. I will give you a very simple answer. It's actually easy.

It's the knowledge.

And the knowledge is pretty simple. It's so easy to go around the roundabout. Why do we over-complicate so many things in life including fitness and food?

Do you think celebrities and models were born under a lucky star or something? Why do you think they hire a personal trainer or a qualified person? You don't have to spend days and years in the gym, but if you do, great. I hope you are having a great time.

What you need to know to be in a good shape, and to have the body you want we can teach you in around 10 hours, but we don't like you to know this as we also need clients.

I will keep this as simple as possible, as I think I might be still confused about 5 a day and all those macronutrients and micronutrients and all this rather complicated stuff. I am also not going to be telling you here how important a healthy life style is ... it's your life.

There was one more thing that amazed me after talking to my clients. We tend to do the roundabouts everywhere, and to be honest, I prefer roundabouts at the gym. At least, you feel great after the workout. The one's in private life drain the soul out of you.

As I am like most people, I had done both types of roundabouts myself. I want to save you little bit of time and energy, and try to give you an exit for both. I am so talented that I had to find psychology books as my roundabouts made me very dizzy. I hope this book will help you, make you smile at what we are as humans and will explain a lot.

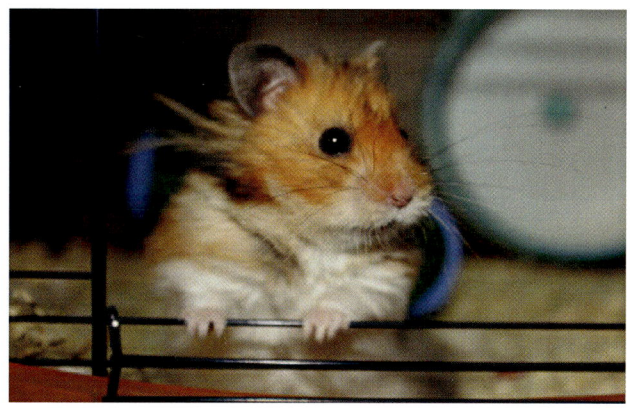

Chapter 1

TAKE THE EXIT & I WILL SURVIVE THIS FAMILY

Home sweet home

Christmas is coming soon, and you are so excited. Maybe you are lucky and have a lovely family! You can't wait for this magical time when everyone gets together when joy, food and love are everywhere.

How wonderful!

Once a year. We are all happy, forget about dieting, and we enjoy the food without guilt or (God help us), feeling the need to count calories. Who would? We eat all this food, lie on the sofa, watch Christmas movies and drink lots of mulled wine. Family time, food and drink bring us so much joy.

Becoming an alcoholic

Not so happy, perhaps you are dreading it! You have been a scapegoat in this narcissistic family since you can remember, and you can't wait for all those stupid arguments where you are not quite sure if you will laugh or cry, especially after a few hours of listening to how amazing everyone is.

You feel like that three glasses of wine will not be enough. To cap it all, here comes that stupid question "why are you still not married?" or "when are you planning to have kids?". Oh yeah! Oh, I forgot to mention that question "when are you going to get a proper job?" or "when are you going to lose some weight?". All so you are seen as acceptable to your family, and they no longer have to pretend that you somehow appeared here by accident.

You only have to hear the word family, and you begin to quiver. After a few hours spent together, you make a trip to the shop, and just to be sure you will be able to cope, you buy all the mulled wine that is on the shelf!

Single again

Another Christmas comes along, and you are still single or maybe single again (left by your boyfriend or girlfriend just before Christmas!). The idea of spending Christmas with your family is horrifying, so indulging in lots of food, drink and ice cream is fantastic!

After the New Year, you will go back to the gym, and you are going to do your best, being single again, this time you're definitely going to meet the love of your life! The better you look, the better the chance someone will ask you out. You are going to nail it this time!

Of course, you will look amazing, and your ex is going to regret he left you, a couple of drunken nights will do for now …

Danger zone

Oh God, this Christmas you have to spend time with your girlfriend's family. You are dreading it. You would love to eat your mother in law, but you can't. You hate the idea of this time together with them. The only thing that is going to keep you sane is food and drink. Of course, then you will be accused of being an alcoholic. Oh, never mind! Still, it's better than looking at those critical faces telling you that you should be doing more of this or that.

You'll buy yourself a couple of bottles of JD that will get you by and keep you happy or maybe sane over the next couple of days.

Somehow you think of this terribly anxious person terrified of flying that needs to have a few drinks beforehand, otherwise he might get a heart attack. You somehow feel the same as he does. Only you would rather see a plane and not your mother in law. You must get drunk too before you even turn up, but of course just like this nervous passenger, you are going to pretend nothing is wrong. Otherwise, they would not let you on board. You secretly open the bottle of JD before you go for the visit and hope that your girlfriend will not notice a thing. God alcohol! Sometimes it is so needed!

It's January

JOLENE …

… is a young female who just turned 30. Her Bf has just left before Christmas, and she is desperately trying to put her life back together. She has always had an abusive family, but she believed that it must be due to her doing something wrong, and the abuse she gets, she somehow deserves. Otherwise, why would they do it?

It's after Christmas, and she is back at the gym! She is fully going back to exercise and working really hard. She is running on the treadmill, and the image of her fat hamster Boris in the running wheel is crossing her mind rather more often than it should.

Back at home, every morning, she performs an athletic jump onto her scales. When she looks at the number she thinks to herself, "a couple of zeros added to this number would look great on my bank account statement, but as my weight!?" Surely it is wrong. She cannot be this heavy, and she does not eat that much. It must be the scales. She is sure it's the scales.

A few days after some more hard work at the gym, she gets home and looks at Boris. He was running before she left for the gym, and he is still running. She wonders if he had a break or not. Why is Boris still fat then? Maybe she feeds him too much, she wonders. But she is struggling to remember if she actually fed him in the last two days?

Boris, the hamster, runs like a maniac in his wheel, and Jolene is making another trip to the gym.

So far, she has mastered her athletic jump onto the weight scales, but now she is convinced that the scales are faulty. Back to the shop, and she buys another set, just to be sure. She even buys the one that sadistically reports her body fat.

The next day, and another athletic jump onto the new scales, but the number is definitely wrong! She is furious. She looks at Boris, and she gets angry as he looks like he is laughing at her while he is running like crazy. She hates the hamster. He even looks like he is enjoying himself running and does not care, he is rather fat! She furiously takes his wheel away from him just to feel better and calms herself down with a glass of her favourite red wine.

The next morning, she goes back to the gym again. After she gets home, she returns the wheel to Boris, and she gives him some food. She removes the scales from the bathroom and tries to forget about her meltdown yesterday. Stay calm and keep on running - everything is going to be just fine, she tells herself.

Awake in the morning, and she tries to convince herself to be positive. She does feel better, and she is sure the scales are faulty. She leaves for work, and as soon as she gets to the office, there is chocolate cake smiling at her. Oh, she forgot that it's Debbie's birthday. She is trying to resist the chocolatey temptation.

Everyone is looking at her and wondering if she will manage to say no or just going to eat it. She eats it, and OMG, it tastes so good! She is having a little moment, as she had been resisting chocolate for a while. The question of which is better, chocolate or sex, is crossing her mind. It then dawns on her that everyone is looking at her because her facial expression is more like she is having an orgasm rather than shoveling chocolate cake into her mouth. She hopes no one notices how much joy she is having at this moment. She is sure these people have no idea what it feels like to resist chocolate for a few weeks. She is hoping no one is going to ask that stupid question, "how's your diet going?"

Back to her desk, and she feels so guilty. She starts thinking about fat Boris again. How come the hamster never gets tired of running? She starts to think about taking his wheel away from him again, just to feel better. She will go back to the gym this evening anyway, and she is going to burn it off. She has it under control, but maybe she should not eat anything else today. Just to be sure. Stay calm, she tells herself.

She goes to the gym. Feeds Boris when she gets back home. The next day she remembers that she is supposed to have dinner and few drinks with friends. She forgot but goes out anyway. Never mind, it's ok. She is going to be good.

She has her first drink and then a second. The diet is completely forgotten, but she is having a great time. After she gets home, she has another drink. The squeaky voice of Boris' wheel reverberates in the flat, and she realises she failed again. She goes to the fridge, and with another glass of wine in her hand, she makes sure she takes out everything edible. She goes to bed with chocolate all over her face and feels so happy and frustrated at the same time before passing out! After getting up in the morning and making a cup of coffee, she is wondering how many people she had over last night as someone cleared out the fridge …

She wonders if Boris should be put on a diet too.

Jolene meets John

Jolene's friend keeps on talking about his boss, and she is curious to meet him. She might end up working with him one day, and he might be her boss. He is successful, managed to get a great position in this large aviation company before forty, while some people try without success for their whole working life. She hears some impressive stories about him, and she thinks to herself that this guy is an interesting character.

She meets him …

After ten minutes, she thinks to herself, "gosh, what a nutter!" She gets angrier and angrier, as he managed to upset her within a few minutes as he sat her down after she offered to buy him a drink. How rude! She wonders how she will be able to keep the conversation going with this guy. She is dreading the fact that she will be sitting there for a couple of hours.

Somehow the night ends up pretty well, and she ends up the next day with a massive hangover, and a couple of unwanted visits to the bathroom. Jolene was impressed by John at the end of the evening and hopes to meet him again at some point.

John has a very stressful job. He spends most of his time in the office, as he ended up just like most of us, on the emotional rollercoaster called marriage.

Frog

She starts to think about the psychological story of a frog. She loves animals even though she has an occasional emotional outburst with Boris when she hides his running wheel.

When you put a frog into boiling water, the frog jumps out. If you put a frog into cold water and gently raise the heat, the frog loses the ability to jump out before noticing how hot the water has got and is boiled to death. Somehow, she feels as if John is in hot water, as he looked exhausted. She is hoping that someone will pull the plug out before this frog dies. This frog is rather different in a nice way.

John

John sits in the office, and his mind wanders off as he is thinking about the upcoming meeting. He opens the drawer and gets the bag of Chocolate Orange chunks out. He starts eating them while he is thinking about how the meeting is going to go. After a while, he puts his hand in, but all the chocolates are gone. Gosh, he hadn't noticed he'd eaten the whole bag. Never mind. He'll buy another one tomorrow morning. Oh no! He won't! He's trying to give up this habit.

The following morning, he buys another bag of chocolates.

As he is in a senior position in the company and Christmas is coming, he ends up going to six Christmas parties. He feels a bit heavy, shall we say? He starts to think that maybe he will buy a hamster for his lovely kids, so the hamster will remind him daily that he should do some exercise. Clearly, he cannot buy a hamster for himself!

John is pretty exhausted, as he has got so much on his shoulders. He can't be bothered with exercise. He is just knackered.

John goes and buys a hamster for his kids.

The hamster exercises daily, and John buys another bag of chocolates on his way to work.

A few weeks later, he buys a new suit as this one is getting tight.

The hamster keeps on running.

John has a lot of pressure to perform at work, and on top of this, he has lots of people that would love to push him off his pedestal. He is familiar with jealousy.

Oh, and I forgot to mention. His boss is a female. He is prone to emotional outbursts, and sometimes he just feels like a Chocolate Orange bag is simply required to keep him sane, even though he gets on with his female boss pretty well.

Jolene is single, and she just met this hot guy

Gosh, he is cute. They exchange a few messages and are planning their first date. She gets home from work and takes her clothes off for a shower. She glances in the mirror and is filled with shock. Or maybe a panic attack, but she doesn't know what a panic attack is, but she guesses it probably feels like this.

She immediately starts to think about the quickest diet on the planet, as her body reminds her of something rather massive, but she can't quite work out what it reminds her of.

She starts to think. Maybe he is not even going to message me again.

She gets out of the shower, and her phone beeps. Jolene is dying of excitement, but in fact, it's her mother reminding her of a family dinner next week. She is dreading her mother's comments about her weight already.

She gets a little anxious and thinks to herself, "he is not going to message me. I am too big". She puts Victoria's Secret lotion on after the shower just to remind herself how those supermodels look, and she ends up banging her head on the fridge door as she is trying to dig out the chocolate she hid so well in the fridge last week, in the hope, that she will forget it's there. But the message from her mother was a great trigger to find something sweet. She needs it.

The next morning, she has a message, and she is dying of excitement as she never believed he would get back to her. He did!

She goes on a diet, again. She must look her best, but she ate so much yesterday she decides the best diet is not to eat anything! She is nearly fainting in the office, but she must make this! This guy seems like her match!

Later on, friends ask her to come out for something to eat, but she makes up some story about an upset stomach as she must not eat! She goes to the gym the same evening, and she is waiting for this guy to message her again.

He doesn't message for days, and she keeps on starving herself and running at the gym. She manages for a couple of days, but when her friends are ready to call an ambulance, she realizes that maybe she should eat again.

She eats, and she eats a lot. What's the point? He doesn't message.

She wakes up in the morning, and there he is! He has messaged again! She cries. In the last few days, she has eaten so much that her weekly food shop has only lasted two days.

She is ready to starve again.

Boris died…

He died fat …

He did lots of exercise ….

Jolene is sure he died of exhaustion.

She goes, and she buys another hamster.

Us humans

Sometimes it's good to laugh, and sometimes it's good to cry. Sometimes it's even great to go a little crazy.

What Jolene and John are experiencing is pretty normal for many of us.

We keep on going around and around. We feel good, then we feel guilty, and then we feel good again. It's not healthy for our bodies, but it's also unhealthy for our mental health, with the stress of work and relationships. Food is supposed to make us happy and relaxed and give us emotions of joy, but mostly we just end up with guilt, frustration, sadness, and anger either with ourselves or with food. A love - hate relationship with food, full of frustration. Up to 90% of people gain their weight back within five years of finishing their diet.

We only feel those positive emotions, such as love, joy, and happiness, for a short period of time before those emotions are replaced with guilt or frustration. If only we could feel positivity and good emotions more often.

Ask any person who has had a breakdown. With many people, guilt played a massive role in it. Food is here to keep this vehicle that we call our body, moving us from place to place. If it was a Ferrari, would you look after it a little better?

If you had a Ferrari, you would occasionally feel great putting your foot down and speeding a little and doing some naughty driving. You can't always eat healthily as it would drive you crazy. We all need to be a little cheeky or naughty, but without feeling bad and just enjoy it. But we are somehow so good at losing the balance.

We get so comfortable and so lazy when we have 'u' turns and roundabouts that even when we complain, we are somehow happy. It is so much easier not to take that exit. We do everything not to make changes, and we are amazing with the word BUT.

It's just easier. And sometimes we need the word BUT, as we are only waiting for a disaster to happen to push us off the roundabout and take the exit.

We just happily go around and around, just like that hamster in the wheel. You even watched your hamster going so fast that when he stopped running, the wheel's inertia gave him a few spins around without him putting any effort. You watched him, and you were amazed he did not fly out from his wheel, but he just managed to run like crazy the moment the momentum was gone, without a blink. Somehow watching your hamster reminded you of your life.

You think to yourself, steady she goes ….

But in fact, this is flat out …

We often look for something that will replace emotions, so we use food and addictions, or maybe we look for something that is going to keep our emotions under control.

Emotions and feelings are strong triggers for food choices. We have created a toxic relationship with food, and we have got stuck on the roundabout. Sometimes even in relationships, a little argument is good, but when it's toxic, you might end up like the frog that has lost the ability to jump out after the heat has gone up …

We have so much information and choices that we become frustrated and confused over what's good and what isn't. Food has become a fashion, obsession, or something we need to feel better about ourselves, but the joy has gone.

If I asked you an hour after your lunch how your food tasted, would you be able to answer with a smile on your face, or rather frustration as if the lunch was something stressful? Do you even remember if you enjoyed your lunch? Do you go for lunch and you have mixed feelings as you feel like you can't wait to have some food but are dreading the fact that later you are going to think to yourself, "I wish I ate a little less"? Or "I wish I had had more self-control and had a salad"?

Hemingway used to describe how his food tasted. In his book, A Moveable Feast, he writes of eating oysters. He suggests that eating is about more than getting, preparing and consuming food.

"As I ate oysters with their strong taste of the sea and their faint metallic taste that the cold white wine washed away, leaving only the sea taste and succulent texture, and as I drank their cold liquid from each shell and washed it down with the crisp taste of the wine, I lost the empty feeling and began to be happy and to make plans."

"We ate well and cheaply and drank well and cheaply and slept well and warm together and loved each other."

"Drinking wine was not a snobbism nor a sign of sophistication nor a cult; it was as natural as eating and to me as necessary.

A Moveable Feast by Ernest Hemingway

We have lost the joy, and many of us are like a hamster running like crazy. But the hamster might have more fun than we do.

I will explain some tricks we can use, how I do it as I am very familiar with 'u'-turns. Once you gain the knowledge, things will be so much easier for you and understanding what is happening and gaining more self-awareness will bring more joy into your life. I hope you will find joy in food and your body.

Why U-turns and roundabouts

Many of us suffer from a lack of self-love. We are addicted to unhappiness and to an unhealthy roundabout, constantly chasing something that will eventually, we hope, make us happy.

Were you raised in a family where arguments were a daily occurrence? Maybe your parents were so busy arguing that your needs were not met as much as you needed. Psychologists say that 86% of families are dysfunctional. We all have some emotional scars, and *food* can sometimes help us cope and help us feel good, but frankly, we should experience food as Hemingway did.

Maybe you have adopted your parents' habits when it comes to food, and maybe you used chocolates and sweets as a pleasant escape when your parents were having a battle.

Maybe you felt lonely as a child, and food was giving you comfort.

Maybe you were bullied, and food was making you feel good.

Or is it just too comfortable to get stuck at the roundabout?

Sometimes getting off the roundabout can make us feel we are losing something of value, and we fear that we won't be able to adapt to new ways. It can feel like a threat to our safety and security, as we are so familiar with our ways that something new and unknown can be scary. We might also become scared of admitting to ourselves that our coping patterns were wrong and unhealthy; it threatens our safety deep inside. We can become scared that we will be unable to maintain new habits.

It can feel as if we have lied to ourselves for so long, and suddenly we have to face our lies, which can be pretty emotional. We can be driven by fear of seeing the truth of what drives us towards unhealthy habits and unhealthy roundabouts.

After making changes, we can also become angry with ourselves for not having made changes earlier, but we need to remember it's better late than never.

You might be addicted to this up and down roller coaster you are on, as you have been stuck in this situation for so long, you are used to it. And you are subconsciously seeking it, even if it's unhealthy for your body and soul.

You might have to look inside and answer this for yourself. Why you keep on going around in circles, and why it is so difficult to take the exit? If it's just the knowledge, I am more than happy to help you out with your food roundabouts.

I am going to show you how we take the exit from the roundabout when it comes to food, weight loss and our body. I am going to show you a few psychological roundabouts you might not know about. But I am not going to go too deep as I am not a qualified psychologist, but I want to show you that talking to a qualified person is sometimes the best thing you can do. I am going to explain to you how things work, don't work, and how simple it is when it comes to food and weight loss. When you have the knowledge, you are winning.

FOR THE SOUL ...

I WILL SURVIVE THIS FAMILY

The scapegoat in a narcissistic family pattern

Many people are lucky in life and have supportive families. And it is a blessing. Many people have families, but they might have felt their whole life as if they simply don't belong to this family. They feel a little anxious the moment when they open social media and see all those comments about how the family is everything. For many people, family is a source of suffering. Those people might have heard of the term scapegoat in a narcissistic family pattern. I am writing this book to bring a little more knowledge on mental health, as many people are struggling these days, and many people will experience some psychological problems through life. I am hoping that this little extra knowledge is going to be helpful, and when someone is experiencing a problem, they look into books about healing, as it's important to look after the body and the soul.

Who is a scapegoat

Generally, the person who tells the truth in a family system. Because of truth – telling, this person became a target for lies, manipulations and anger from the family.

The scapegoat in a narcissistic family is usually the strongest, nicest, most empathetic person, and it makes them dangerous, as they reveal the truth as they can see through the bullshit.

Sometimes the scapegoat needs to leave the family as the abuse becomes unbearable.

Scapegoats have a tendency to have self-doubts throughout life but are often the sanest people.

The type of people who became problem solvers and become targets for narcissistic people, as narcissistic abuse is familiar to them, and they can be subconsciously looking for narcissistic relationships as they are familiar to them. Scapegoats are people with empathy towards others. They tend to look after others but tend to look after others while putting themselves second. It leads to depression.

Strengths of a scapegoat

independent thinker

strong - willed person

empathetic

justice - seeking

emotionally reactive

sensitive

protective of others

caregiving

different in some ways

One of the best things a scapegoat from a narcissistic family can do is find a therapist or self-help psychology books to help with their healing. There is the possibility of hidden emotional traumas from childhood, which can lead to unhealthy behaviour patterns in adulthood and lead to further emotional traumas.

These people are usually lovely in their nature, but because of a tendency to self-doubt, they sometimes get used and abused by narcissistic people, leading to more traumatic events.

These people can quite often feel as if they never belonged to their family and, as someone once said: "I was accidentally born into this family."

Other indicators you might been scapegoated

You might identify as being *co-dependent, highly sensitive* or *empathetic*. You might people please in order to avoid conflict.

You might have difficulty expressing your feelings as you have learned this can be used against you.

If you have been told very often that you are *cold, unloving, selfish, dramatic* by someone close or by a parent.

You might struggle with addictions, depressions, anxiety, co-dependency, obsessive compulsive behaviours due to abuse.

Every time your relationships go wrong, you tend to blame yourself. You feel responsible for your relationship with your parents. Everything is always viewed as your fault.

Often being labelled *crazy, mental, mad, mentally ill* or *emotionally ill* by close members of the family.

You have been emotionally, physically, sexually abused, gaslighted and things were twisted, so the abusers were shown in a better light at your expense?

You have been labelled as *difficult*, a *liar*, *dramatic* or *sensitive*?

You feel there is something innately wrong with you in your adult life, and you are somehow different.

The moment you are supposed to see the family members or go home, you feel uneasy, anxious, or even sick, but you cannot explain why.

You might have difficulty trusting people, forming healthy attachments, trusting loving relationships and friendships, and being more attracted to addicts, narcissists, abusers and continue to form damaging relationships. It all feels like a roundabout.

Therapy and medication might help, but not much.

You don't feel emotionally safe around people.

You always feel more like a punch bag or a door mat.

You might also be labelled the black sheep of the family.

You are having dark thoughts and never feel good enough.

Many scapegoats become successful problem - solvers, carers and are very special people, but they are not aware of it, as self-doubt and self-loathing have crept up inside and never left.

What might happen if you mention to your (narcissistic) family that you are seeking therapy? You might be attacked, as some unhealthy people need scapegoats, as it's beneficial for them to have someone else being attacked and not themselves. Also, many members of the family will feed their ego by giving you kicks, and some cannot see how nasty they are. They feel power. If you change and won't accept the abuse any more, they might be angry, as they benefited from you being a scapegoat. A possible answer from the family is that you are crazy and need therapy, hoping it will discourage you from going (as they might be scared you will find out they have the personality disorder), or they will say that you don't need therapy as you are what you are and stop complaining as the family is only trying to help you out, and you are ungrateful.

Help

Number of books and YouTube videos.

YouTube videos: Dr Ramani and Les Carter PhD

https://bit.ly/3elzPzn

https://youtu.be/v6A9cR93MNU

Book: When pleasing you is killing me by Les Carter PhD

There are many YouTube videos of just 10-15 minutes from both of them.

Therapy that helps with emotional traumas: EMDR, Cognitive behaviour therapy.

Narcissistic abuse can drive many people to have suicidal thoughts. The abuse is hidden and manipulative. The narcissist is a master in gaslighting.

Remember that the narcissist always needs a target, and a scapegoat is needed. The book "Gaslight Effect" also talks very well about not joining the tango dance, where you are drawn back into the narcissist's dance.

Once you know what the label is, it's easy to find support groups where people talk about their journey and healing.

Many psychologists don't like to use labels, as many victims get labels applied to them wrongly by their abusers.

Once you realise that many beliefs you had towards yourself were put there intentionally by narcissists, you can start working on healing. You will learn to know yourself, your true self. You will be surprised, as it's a beautiful journey, but it can be painful.

Many scapegoats are beautiful souls inside and out, but they can't see their own value.

Finding a therapist you connect with can also be challenging, but the moment you find the right one, you will be pleased you made an effort. Some books might be beneficial to read first, as some therapists can also be narcissistic themselves. These books will give you red flags if you should meet one with narcissistic tendencies.

The books will give you a greater understanding, as some therapists are not educated on narcissism. Also, look for qualified people when looking for help. Friends and family are great, but sometimes they can make things worse for you as they cannot see the emotional damage.

You are a human being with emotions, and they were hit badly.

You are not crazy, mental, mad or emotional. You are going for a sanity check if you finally decide to talk to a professional.

"Narcissistic personality disorder is the only illness where the patient doesn't end up in the therapy, but everyone else around does."

Positives if you were a scapegoat

You can heal. You have the power of enjoying and experiencing freedom. You are not scared of being alone. You have felt like this most of your childhood. Scapegoats from narcissistic families, once healed, are strong individuals. You can adapt to situations as you can change easily compared to people from more stable families.

You might become an individual with high emotional intelligence and self-awareness. Scapegoats from narcissistic families are independent thinkers and often smart people as they became scapegoats because of their ability to see the nonsense. They can live lonely lives but are very emotionally intelligent people.

Books and therapy are a great way of understanding the dynamics in narcissistic families and restoring the self-worth that has been damaged by narcissistic abuse.

Once you know you have been a scapegoat, you have a great chance to see your strengths and benefit from them. Remember, you might not even know you have hidden emotional traumas, but at some point in life, when met with a traumatic event, those feelings can come to light and overwhelm you. Then might be the time to find a therapist, but if you do it before meeting a traumatic life event, you are giving yourself more time to live an emotionally satisfying life with healthy self-love.

Being abused is not your fault, but it is your responsibility to seek help for healing yourself.

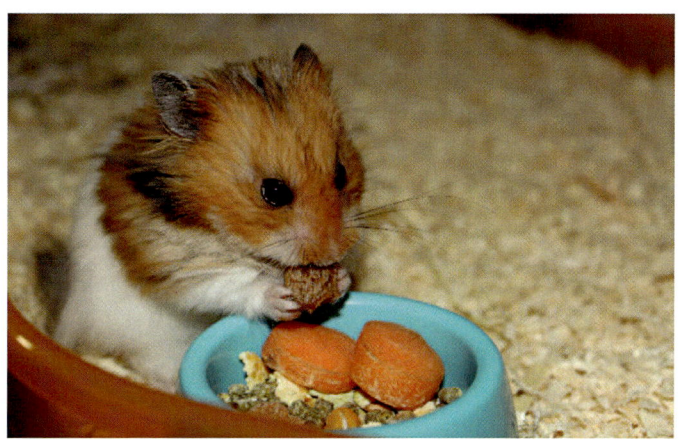

Chapter 2

CRAZY EMOTIONS & ENOUGH IS ENOUGH

Humans and emotions

Aren't we emotional? Well, most of us are. Ask a person who has been through an emotional breakdown, and they will talk for hours about what emotions can do to you. Hopefully, they managed to recover, and once they tell you about their emotional outbursts, it will be with a smile on their face.

It can be hard.

Jolene gets emotional just watching the hamster!

She watches the hamster being fed. He shovels the food first into his left cheek, as much as he can, and then into his second cheek, as full as possible. His front teeth are out as he has got so much food in, he can't close his mouth. He looks so happy with so much food in his mouth he even looks like he is smiling.

Oh well.

After Christmas Jolene is back at the gym, and she has got herself another hamster, Boris. She is full of emotions like everyone else, and so sure this year she will not fail, and she will get her dream body.

The gym is so full that she feels more like it's a night out in a club where everyone sweats, having consumed large amounts of alcohol before throwing in the dance moves to impress someone, but it's not.

It's the gym.

She desperately tries to look like she knows exactly what she is doing, so no one notices her doubting if this will actually work. She gets on the running machine, and all she can think about is food and what she is going to eat for dinner, without guilt, after she gets home. Not many healthy things are crossing her mind. She starts to dream of pizza! No! Run! Run faster! Just like Boris. If he can, I can!

It's mid - Feb.

She is still running. More than ever and faster than ever. At least that's what she thinks. She gets home, and she performs her usual athletic jump on the scales. She doesn't know if she should smile or cry. She has lost 2kgs since Christmas, but she has been running for the last month and a half like Forest Gump, and she swears she can compete against Boris for speed and how much faster her legs are moving, but so much running and only 2 kgs? Well, I guess it's better than nothing, but how much more running have I got to do to get to my dream weight?

Oh, hang on! I did not shave my legs for a week; she gets excited! Maybe if I shave them, it's going to be another kg! She gets emotional again.

She hides the scales.

She returns to her room, where another set of scales is looking at her, so she pushes them so far under the bed that they will be difficult to find.

It's been exhausting.

She is wondering if she feels any good after all this time at the gym or rather depressed. She hears squeaks behind her coming from Boris' spinning wheel. She is starting to get angry, and her emotions go through the roof, so she decides to hide the hamster too. Only for a day.

She feels a little down, but she starts to Google miracle diets while at work and finds one! She gets a boost! This diet works! She feels full of hope after reading all the reviews. After another session at the gym where she sweated hard, she gets home and pulls the hamster out from the wardrobe where she had hidden the poor thing and she digs out the scales from under her bed.

She is ready to start.

Start again!

The first week on a new diet, and she has lost a kg! She is so happy but somehow a little doubtful. She is doing everything right, but two weeks later, her scales shows her that she has put a kg back on!

She gets angry.

She thinks to herself.

"Maybe I am jumping on the scales with too much force?" She gently steps back from the scales, and she steps on them again, this time like a ballerina, thinking she is as light as a feather.

Her weight is the same, and she gets furious! She hides everything again, including Boris, and her next visit is the fridge! She opens it up, and she realizes there is nothing in there that can make her feel better! She orders a take-away, and of course, a bottle of wine! Oh, she has not felt this emotional for a while! She feels great after finishing the pizza and a bottle of her favourite wine.

She goes to bed.

In the morning, she searches for the hamster, but he is nowhere to be found. She starts to worry whether she threw him out of the window, but she is too scared to look. She has to go to work. She opens the door and trips over the cage with the hamster. She had put the poor thing behind the door. She feels embarrassed and a bit guilty, hoping no one saw him out there. Well, if anything, she will say the neighbour tried to take him.

When she gets home from work, she still feels a little emotional, she goes around the house, and this time hides all the mirrors she can find. No one needs to have mirrors in the house! I know what I look like, thank you, she rambles on to herself.

She watches her favourite City of Angels in the evening, and she does not bother with the gym. She sees the heart rate monitor on the TV, and she is watching it going up and down and up and down and then it stops. Somehow, she has a similar feeling right now, as she feels mentally exhausted from this rollercoaster ride. The only thing that is not exhausted is the hamster.

BROKEN

Ellie is in her late thirties and has just suffered a breakdown after splitting up with her fiancée. But she does not know she has had a nervous breakdown.

She nearly ended up running over this idiot on a bicycle who called her stupid after trying to be polite to him.

She is sitting in her car and wondering what the heck just happened as her emotions went through the roof and never returned to normal.

Gosh, she cannot quite work out why she flipped so much, as she has been called far worse in her life, but this guy was an idiot. She sits there, and she drives to the nearest petrol station as she needs to do something or move as she is still absorbing the shock. As she walks in, she sees Ritter sports chocolate bars on the shelves with different flavours. She buys six of them. One of each flavour, as somehow this makes her feel better. Would I feel better if I had run him over? I probably would, she wonders out loud!

She sits in her car, and she opens the first bar of chocolate. She feels sorry for herself. A few weeks back, her ex fiancée got married to someone else on her planned wedding date, and she starts crying. She wonders how much he must have hated her, to do something like this.

She opens a second strawberry flavoured chocolate bar. She wonders how much better she would feel if she had managed to run the idiot over that called her stupid.

She starts to think that maybe she should buy herself a pet as she feels so lonely. Maybe a hamster?

She opens the third bar with weird yoghurt taste, and she cannot be sure if it tastes delicious or disgusting. She feels sick. She cries again.

She feels better.

Suddenly she is terrified! She realises she still has the baseball bat in the car she bought when she was terrified of a psychotic lodger. Her landlord had moved him in and told her he is shy. He was like a chameleon in a jungle, changing his behaviour depending on who was around. He was anything but shy! Oh well. Maybe I am crazy, she whispers to herself. She realises how lucky this guy was, as if she had remembered, he might have ended up with a baseball bat stuck in his head. She has no idea she is experiencing an emotional breakdown and keeps on crying and screaming at people like crazy.

She drives home and keeps on crying. She managed to eat all six chocolate bars on her way home. At least it made her feel like she is doing something, and somehow, it's relaxing. She walks into the house. When her friend sees her, she is terrified!

What happened!?

She walked in with a face looking like a tomato as she is very fair skinned, and she managed to cry for a few hours, with sad mascara streaks on her cheeks, chocolate all over her mouth and a baseball bat in her hand!

I nearly killed some guy as he called me stupid, she responds to her friend.

With a baseball bat, her friend shouts? No! I forgot I had it in my car!

Thank god for that, she replies! I'll get you a drink. You look like you need one!

She says thanks and is desperately trying to work out what to do with the baseball bat. She is terrified as she is losing control over her emotions, and it's scary. Chocolate makes her feel good.

What drives us?

Have you ever wondered who you are? What drives you? Why you behave the way you do? Has stress or emotional or physical trauma changed you or someone you know?

What drives you, and what emotions are you craving? What do you do when your emotional needs are not met? Is it love or fear that drives you? They are two feelings with strong emotional responses, and many people are driven by one or the other without being aware. Many people are driven by money, power, ego, sex, and when their emotional needs are not met, many people succumb to addictions, alcohol, abusive substances, cigarettes, sugar, food, MSG. You can be addicted to complaining, unhappiness, sadness, an abusive partner, and not realising the toxic relationship you are in.

Food industry and emotions

Ok, let's be serious for a while. You have probably noticed where I am going with this. Humans are very emotional, and the food industry is aware of this. Humans have addictive tendencies. Maybe not even that. We like things that make us feel good.

Have you noticed that exercise is at first painful, but later, after exercise, you feel great? When it comes to food, most food makes us feel great first and a little later, much worse than before. But because of this and other factors, when you feel bad, you are not going to start doing push-ups, but you go and buy whatever makes you feel great, and as quickly as possible. We would all look like supermodels and love our bodies if it was the other way round.

We have so much stress and do so much for everyone else that food becomes our only happiness source. As we get stressed, we start looking for things that give us quick and positive emotions. Food is amazing in these terms; it gives you exactly this.

It would be great if when we feel bad, we could immediately have sex with someone we truly love and feel a rush of beautiful emotions and excitement, but again they don't sell it in the shops and having those kinds of relationships can be so rare. Many people feel like they have been emotionally starved for a very long time. We have to wait for these kinds of relationships, but maybe the longer we wait, the better it gets when we finally find what our soul was looking for. Sometimes a very long time. That's why we have chocolate!

Let's have a look at how the Food Industry works

Business…

As long as the product is sold with the right profit margin, it is considered doing well. We all want something. We have emotions. We want to feel good, loved, needed. Sometimes we are missing something, so instead of looking deep down for what's missing, we create a strong relationship with food or another addiction.

The food industry knows how to give people the emotions that they are craving. They spend millions and millions on how to create the most addictive products. People are hooked on their products, so they are getting sales, making profits, and you are somehow happy in the short term. And because it's only for the short term, you want it again and again and again.

Thanks to these many addictions, we lose our balance, and food becomes the factor that makes us happy. Pay attention to how you feel. Maybe you needed to fulfil your emotions, and you used food to achieve that. The food industry is very clever, and they use chemicals to support this. Sugar is much more addictive than cocaine.

People going through or close to burn out (psychologists say every fifth person is going to experience burn out) are experiencing an emotional response, perhaps with physical exhaustion, and food can be a tremendous sticking plaster for many things.

Some people can gain lots of weight going through this, and on the other hand, some can lose a lot, as they become so stressed, feel sick, and struggle to eat.

Emotions, food and additives are linked together.

Attachments to food, like any other attachments which are not healthy, can make you feel like they are sucking the life out of you. It's occupying your mind more than it should.

Some people spend their whole day thinking about what to eat to lose weight. Their thoughts become obsessive, and they spend far too much time thinking about food.

The moment we are not happy with our weight and how we look, we start to think about food. This makes us eat even more for comfort, or we starve ourselves. It's easy for us to become addicted to food.

Sometimes the number shown on the scales can become our indicator of happiness. The food industry is very aware of how humans think. Unfortunately, the other side effects are not as important, so long as the food companies are making a profit.

Artificial sweeteners

Used in over 6,000 products in our food shops.

Aspartame is sold under other names such as NutraSweet, Equal, and Spoonful. The American Food and Drug Administration has received more complaints about Aspartame than any other additive in history. Aspartame was previously listed as a biochemical warfare agent!

Many people with diabetes use this drug. It is found in sugar free beverages, power bars, low calorie soft drinks, some chewable VITAMIN supplements and some of these products are labelled as 'health products' such as diet sodas. Yes, 6000 products.

Sweeteners used in the food industry are thought by some experts to cause brain stimulation and potentially craving sensations and appetite.

Side effects of sweeteners and additives

Seizures, dizziness, blurred visions, hallucinations, headaches, depression. Other symptoms listed are muscle spasm, WEIGHT

GAIN, rashes, nausea, breathing difficulties, anxiety attacks, LOSS OF TASTE, vertigo, memory loss, joint pain, and I can go on and on and on…….and yes, this drug is in 6,000 products available to consumers. Weight gain and loss of taste. I will talk later about how your taste cells are affected by these drugs.

Sugar and the immune system response

Our brains have short term memory, and we remember that we felt great. So, we crave that feel good moment again. Who would not?

Sugar and junk food can produce a burst of energy and can give you those emotions of comfort in the short term. Short term solutions. We can call it the pain-killer effect of sugar that comes from the release of endorphins in your body when you eat sugar. Endorphins are morphine like chemical that naturally circulates in your body when you exercise or are excited or eat sweet, salty or spicy food. But despite how you feel and how great it is, sugar has a dramatic effect on your immune system for hours after consumption. That's the price for it.

When you eat sugar, it directly competes with your immune cells and with Vitamin C. More sugar, less space for Vitamin C in your immune system. The result is a weakened defence against infections.

We naturally crave sugar. Even human breast milk is sweet.

I could write a whole book on additives, chemicals and sugar, but that's not my intention. I chose to talk about sweeteners and additives because I want to bring to your awareness LOSS OF TASTE.

I like this one, as I have personally experienced it. Think about the food that you eat. Do you often eat the same type of food? What food is it? As you can see, the food industry is using additives and chemicals to create addiction, which makes you buy the same food repeatedly. But what these chemicals do, they numb your taste cells. It's more your brain craving food than your body.

Knowledge is for the brain and experience is for your body.

Here is a little test that works well with many of my personal training clients to make you aware of how your brain is set up for addictions.

You are at work or home, and you are craving chocolate or a binge of salty food. There is a great trick that works with pretty much everyone. Let's say your cravings are getting out of control, and you would kill for sugar. Set your timer for 20 minutes and make yourself wait.

The brilliant result is that 90% of people, after *20 minutes,* are happy to give it a miss. This will make you realize how addictions work. But try to be aware of yourself and what is going on in your brain, how you are thinking and how strong the cravings are. The more you become aware, the more it will be easier to understand yourself and control cravings.

Let's say that it did not work for you, and you had that chocolate or whatever it was you were craving. Let's say it was chocolate. So next time when you try this exercise, all you do is have nearby a strong 80% or 90% cocoa chocolate. Something that you cannot eat all at once as it's too rich. So, you wait for a few minutes and after, let's say, 5-10 minutes, you have a piece of this rich chocolate. The craving will become less and less after a few minutes, and you won't have a need for whatever you were craving.

Later on, I will give you examples of clean eating but what I want to stress is that the more cleanly you eat, the more your taste buds are going to come back, and food will start to taste different, in fact much nicer and richer. Some people are more aware of this, and some are less. Everyone is different.

Other issues we are facing are stress eating, emotional eating, comfort eating and others…. Most of the stories I gave you in the first chapter were of emotional eating or stress eating.

Food is an anxiety treatment.

A psychologist friend of mine mentioned that addiction to sugar can be a replacement for love.

Have a think about it.

One more thought for you

Did you know these days after we die, the body struggles to dissolve itself compared to 50 years back? During our lifetime, our body becomes a chemical tin that can last for a very long time. Use common sense. You planted tomatoes in your garden. After the harvest, how long do your tomatoes remain edible?

Not long, is it? How long can you eat tomatoes from a tin, five years after canning? Now imagine what it does to your body.

FOR THE SOUL…

ENOUGH IS ENOUGH!!!

Many people will, unfortunately, experience burnout, emotional breakdown or a nervous breakdown.

Why do people end up having a breakdown? Well, I was told by a psychologist it's pretty simple. None of us knows our limit, and we keep telling ourselves that we are ok and can do it. And we do too much, and sometimes we have to, but we do not realize we are reaching our limit, and then it can be too late. (frog story …)

Sometimes our bodies are giving us signals, but we are good at ignoring these as we simply don't have the time or energy because we are either too busy or stressed out. We push the signal away, and one day our body tells us it's had enough and cannot cope anymore.

It's simply too much. There's too much stress or tiredness (mental or physical), and in many cases, both. Your body has had enough and lost its ability to protect you against stress and pressure. The breakdown will lead to an inability to function normally.

Each breakdown is different from person to person, but the signs are common in responding to prolonged stress and losing the ability to function. Usually, a person will experience emotional, behavioural or physical symptoms. The person can behave completely out of character. It's terrifying for the person experiencing it and can be for people whom involved.

A person's breakdown can be result of having years of too many responsibilities at work and home. For some, it can be a sudden tragedy such as the loss of a partner or another emotional trauma. People who have cared too much for others and put themselves second may experience emotional fatigue, and people with poor boundaries that had not learnt better self care might also end up with an emotional breakdown.

Untreated depression, an anxiety disorder, or panic attacks can finally cause psychotic symptoms if a person is experiencing complete exhaustion. Many people who tend to sweep things under the carpet or, as we say, put it into the "f..k it" box might experience many symptoms as many things are suddenly jumping out at them as if a Pandora's box was opened.

A Road to Recovery

You might have been through a series of traumas and not managed to recover fully, then suddenly you are experiencing a new one. Life tends to throw out more than one trauma at the same time. Maybe you had prolonged and overwhelming stress, traumatic events or challenging life events that required much more time and energy, and you were ok through all of these traumas. You thought to yourself that it's all ok, but unfortunately, our body keeps a stress score. And there is a possibility that one day you will snap, as it is just too much.

If you are asking yourself how long the recovery will take, it depends.

Recovery and what to expect

I'm not going to lie, and it's going to be tough. There are going to be lots of ups and downs and periods of stagnation. The first three months can be difficult. After some time, you will slowly start to feel some sense of normality. If you're going to take antidepressants and medication, be prepared to experience some side effects. You might struggle with your energy levels, and some days you're going to feel much better and some worse. It can be a rollercoaster ride.

When you have a specialist that you can call anytime, it's a big help and will speed up your recovery. You will learn how to put yourself first and look after your well-being as a priority. The quicker you find professional support and help, the faster your recovery is going to be.

When looking for a specialist, remember not every therapist will suit you. If you feel the one you have is not empathetic, or you don't click, go and find yourself a different one. It's your time, and you need the best you can get. It's your life, your body and by caring too much for others, you might have ended up in this position, so remember, this time, it's about you. Be picky.

This was a free fall without a parachute, but you survived it.

Positive outcomes of a breakdown

The chaos will be gone. You will learn healthier coping patterns. Your spiritual consciousness will rise.

You will return to your normal level of functioning and more. You will operate at a higher level than ever before. Remember, if you are down and at your lowest, the only way is up. What goes down must go up.

You become more aware of your own feelings. Your self - awareness will rise. If you read the right books, you will gain the knowledge for life.

One of the reasons we had a breakdown is that we did not learn to be flexible. This is the opportunity to learn so.

Bend, but don't break.

This will be on your mind for the rest of your life….

The breakdown might lead us to changes we always wanted to do or maybe terminate the relationships that were slowly poisoning our souls, but we felt too bad and guilty to do so before. We might have to learn to stop lying to ourselves.

Self-love will become a joy.

You will feel like you lost yourself for a while but not have found new strength.

It's better to fall and recover than balance on edge for the rest of your life. Maybe you felt like you were in a cage the whole time, but now will be a time to learn how to fly.

You survived this….

Take a breath and start looking at the positives…They are there. You just have to find them. Many people who went through this eventually say, 'Thank God it happened.'

You will be one too.

But you might have to *be patient* for a while …

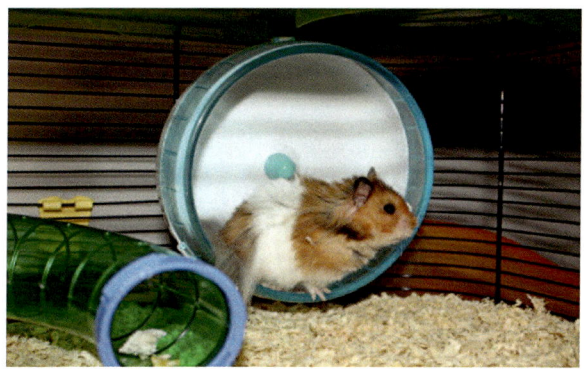

Chapter 3

CAROUSEL NEVER STOPS TURNING & LOSING MY MIND

Eve, if you tell me what to eat, I will eat you too. This message I got from my darling soul sister when she came to me and said I want to lose some weight.

"Look at my belly", she said and started to laugh! "It's big", she shouts and keeps laughing. I love her! I started with a diatribe on what she should do and eat, and after a few minutes, she just rolled her eyes and made her way to switch the oven on. She loves fish! Every night!

She started to prepare her fish, and she stopped listening after five minutes anyway, and all I saw was her excitedly checking the oven with a beaming smile.

The next day I was at the gym, and I finished the session with my client. My phone beeped, and I got a message from her saying, "I will eat you too.".

Roller-coaster ride with diets

Yes, we are weak. We are humans, and we are emotional. Making changes and gaining new habits is almost impossible. Most of us like our routines and the known. We know how we feel, so it keeps us 'safe'. It's nearly impossible to maintain a diet without being grumpy or emotional.

Diets are set up to fail. Why? Because we are addicted to food and when you have a favourite food, and you are not supposed to eat it, you get so grumpy, and you feel like something that you love is missing. Think of a child. When the child is naughty, parents take their favourite toy away, and the child gets emotional. The same happens to you when you stop eating food you like (you take away your pleasure) and replace it with something not so good.

Who wouldn't be emotional?

Love, addictions, feelings, food and emotions are all linked together. Whilst they can feel great, they can be toxic and for humans to maintain balance is sometimes the biggest challenge we can have. I am sure you have been through the rollercoaster ride where you diet like crazy and count every single calorie, almost twice as you are expecting a hot date, but after breaking up, you wipe everything out of the fridge, and nothing in the house escapes. For days you go crazy with ice cream, chocolate and whatever you love. You replace love with food as it just feels great at that moment, as it also helps you forget about the heartache, anxiety, sadness and possibly anger.

Diets are the standard way you will lose a bit of weight, but mentally it's too difficult, so people go back to their old habits. But because they lost a bit of weight, they are thinking to themselves, I am going to go on this diet again as it worked and I lost a few pounds, but this time I am going to be strict with myself, and I am going to make it. It's a crazy roundabout. You could end up for years going forwards and backwards!

A diet becomes your life sentence.

90% of people within 5 years get their original weight back and make a U-turn back to their original habits? The familiar feeling of the *original* is too strong. Remembering those happy feelings that food gave them. They were fat, but they were "happy".

With a diet, all that is going to happen to you is your focus is going to be on food and the number on the scales. The joy, excitement, and positive feelings food once gave you will be put on hold as the focus will be on what you look like, and the number on the scales will be an indicator of your happiness. How grumpy and miserable you will be is another story. You will be excitedly telling people that you are on this diet, and you've lost a few pounds, but deep inside, you hate it, and you are scared; will you have the strength to keep your appetite under control?

Mentally you are trying to avoid the thought that you are lying to yourself, and maybe you are scared deep inside that it will work, and the number, which is the indicator of your happiness, won't make you happy ...

Many people end up on diets that taste horrible, drink shakes, and eat artificial food as they hope for the best. Some even feel a little sick after some (magic) food that will give them the *Bingo* number.

Think about your attitude towards food after a relationship break-up. Many people either eat more, some hardly anything, and some start to drink more than they did before the break-up. Many people use food, alcohol, drugs or just go crazy in the gym purely to forget about those heightened emotions and feelings.

Love and food are two things we crave that we need for our body and soul.

How do you function, and what are your food patterns when you suffer emotional or mental stress?

That idiotic question I used to get when I worked at the gym

<u>Do you ever eat?</u> "No, I live off air!" I used to answer. Well, I am a qualified personal trainer, it would be a little odd if I was overweight, don't you think? Usually, it was someone who was there twice a day and still looked like they badly needed the gym. But I guess we all have to answer some idiotic questions sometimes in our lives. Maybe those people think it's healthy to keep our blood pressure a little higher.

Replacing missing emotions and many other things that are great in life with food is a little silly, but we've all done it!

So … we look for second best.

Sometimes we forget to love ourselves enough and end up believing that if we had that fantastic body, someone would love us a lot more; that might be true, but the soul will suffer.

It's that crazy roundabout, and exiting can be challenging, so keeping a comfortable feeling and those old habits (as they occasionally worked) seems to be the best shot.

We might also be scared of the unknown and possible failure.

When you get the body you wanted, you realize that many things are just a *mind matter, which is; self-love, relationships and our roundabouts*. Understanding your soul can be hard work. How often do you ask yourself, "why do I feel like this?". And when you do, do you know the answer?

The moment you understand how to get to your optimum weight, your crazy roundabout with diets and food will be sorted. This will give you a chance to focus on your mental wellbeing, as your weight and food won't occupy your mind more than needed.

No wonder so many people have anxiety these days and many more mental health problems. Everything becomes artificial, even our own feelings are artificial as we make ourselves feel like this. We look with our eyes, but our souls suffer. We are told many times that something is good for us, and we don't even have enough energy left to challenge whether it is good or not. Then we artificially start feeling it's good even though it might not be good for us at all. We lie to ourselves. But maybe we forget to ask our soul what it is yearning for.

Maybe the crazy roundabout with diets is so exhausting that it's creating an unhealthy balance in our brain and body, and then it becomes exhausting. Are we then addicted to this exhausting roundabout?

Your brain can create an addiction to ups and downs. If you have an addiction, ask people with heavy addictions how difficult it is to get off the roundabout. It's nearly impossible without having someone qualified by your side.

Many people advise meditation. When you switch the roundabout off and your brain can start processing information, you will be more aware of your feelings when you are out of it. Your brain sometimes wants you to switch off as it needs to process information and send you signals of what is good or bad in terms of emotions and feelings.

But how often we ignore it!

However, with around 60 000 thoughts a day, your brain needs you to give it a break for a few minutes every day. In many countries, a power nap is a very popular way to increase brain function. All you do (mostly midday) is just close your eyes for ten minutes and have a power nap. It improves brain function, resulting in better physical and cognitive performance, boosts productivity and alertness, improves memory and learning and elevates mood.

Scientifically proven - what diets do to our souls

Diets come with a whole host of negative effects, apart from being more obsessive and preoccupied around food. Lower self - esteem, lower confidence, depression, sadness, guilt, feeling of failure, higher stress levels, fatigue, nervousness, anxiety, nausea, lower sex appetite, loneliness.

Many people would rather stay at home than go out or meet friends for something to eat. The worst one? You are grumpy all day. Are you now addicted to being grumpy or miserable? Why is it so important what we look like, but not whether we are happy inside?

Around 70% of people spend most of their lives being unhappy in their body or keep on dieting. I could not be bothered to do this!

I want to live life.

And when you think about it, most people are unhappy in their bodies, so their thinking is going to be negative or sad. Then they grab the food that makes them feel good again. Short term, of course, can you see how easy it is to start over-eating? You keep craving those good feelings food is giving you.

There is a lot written about loving one's self and sugar being a replacement. No wonder the soul suffers, and people end up with mental health problems.

This emotional, unhealthy rollercoaster ride becomes so toxic for the body and mind that one eventually becomes ill, either mentally or physically. The toxic stress hormones are permanently winning, and feelings of satisfaction, love, and happiness are a distant memory.

Stress becomes an addiction, just as unhealthy food does, and we wonder why we become ill. Unfortunately, many people don't even realize they are permanently stressed as this state of mind and body becomes a norm for them.

They are happy to be unhappy.

Your day and your metabolism

You wake up in the morning. Well, you are kind of awake. You have a couple of kids, a dog that is a little bonkers with some mental issues (at least that's what you think) and a cat.

Times, when you had lots of sex and lots of energy are a distant memory. These days you pass out watching TV at 8 o'clock with the kids laughing at you and your wife waking you up to go to bed as she can't hear the TV because you are snoring. Your kids are still full of energy, and you love your bed time whilst they seem like their energy levels come from high energy batteries, and you wish they had an off switch and would just go to bed.

You get up in the morning, and you are trying to be organized. The kids are running around like lunatics, and you are trying to catch them to put some clothes on them. You trip over the cat, and the crazy dog is running behind you like a maniac, thinking it's a great game!

You are exhausted. Your wife is yelling at you, as you totally forgot everything she was telling you to do yesterday, and you wonder how you will survive your boss and a couple of meetings today. All you can think of to save you is to put some match sticks in your eyes to keep them open.

So far, the dog has managed to rip your trousers as he was hysterically chasing you around the house and pulling on your trouser legs. You would love to strangle the dog, but the kids would kill you, so you make yourself a strong coffee and make your way to work. The day hasn't even started, and you are exhausted.

You survive your day with 7 strong black coffees and are wondering what to do so the kids get tired really soon, and you can make your way to bed as early as possible. Late night pleasures with your wife are a distant memory, and you are not sure who is more exhausted, you or your wife. You feel like you have been sleepwalking through the last couple of years.

But you are surviving.

Guess who else had to go to 'work' today? Your metabolism. And it 'works' for you and possibly feels the same way as you do. You are the boss. What kind of work have you been throwing at your metabolism?

It's simple. Your metabolism might be just as emotional as you. It might end up with match sticks in its eyes, feet up, asleep, throwing a few tantrums or fuming all day wondering what kind of work this boss is sending its way. What a plonker!

It takes your metabolism about an hour after you wake up to work well. Then it's ready. And it's in best 'work mode' for the day. Just like you in the morning when you start fresh and are ready for the day.

That's why we say to people eat within an hour after waking up. Give it some good work, and it's going to start working full on for the day.

It might start to work, but it's going to be a bit stroppy with you as it's not the kind of "work" your metabolism appreciates, so it's going to start working but not with much enthusiasm.

Or no food came through, so your metabolism is going to put its feet up and do nothing. Your metabolism is most proactive in the morning, and you are the one who is going to set the pace for the coming day.

Just like you, after waking up and working for a couple of hours, your metabolism is getting a little tired and starting to slow down. Your metabolism starts to slow down after 4 hours of work, and then it's ready to work again, but depending on whether work is coming through and what kind of work. If some good work is coming, it gets proactive, but as it has already been working for a couple of hours, it's either going to slow down a little, or keep going with the same pace as you are possibly close to lunchtime. If you give it no work (lunch), it's going to go into sleep mode. Remember, every 4 hours, if you feel a little hungry, your metabolism is working great and fast.

The same happens in a couple of hours into the afternoon, but it's going to be slower as its already worked for a couple of hours, and your body is beautifully clever and memorizes your routine, it *works with you and for you.*

If you have a standard 9-5 job, around about 5'ish, it knows that soon work will finish and it will be time to go home and relax. Around 4 hours before your bedtime, your metabolism is ready to shut down slowly, and if there is more work coming, it can possibly wait for tomorrow, or it's going to be processed very slowly.

Your body and your metabolism + your relationship with your body and food = what you look like ...

Your fat cells

They are your little friends that you don't like. They keep you warm. They protect your organs, *nerves*, looking after your skin, nails and hair. And they are involved in the production of essential hormones in your body.

So, what happens when you start starving them? They go into panic mode and become confused, and refuse to release any more calories. They desperately hold on to any fat you send over, as they are scared there is not enough coming in.

They are trying to save you, as they think, you want to kill the body as your body knows fat is essential to keep you alive. They hold onto any fat in the body like crazy. As no more is coming in, they hold onto the fat like a hamster with food in its mouth.

It becomes an unhealthy and toxic relationship between your fat cells, metabolism and you. You don't give your body what it needs to be happy, and your metabolism and fat cells simply have no idea what is happening.

When you stop feeding your body with fat, cells hold on to any stored fat like crazy and refuse to release any out. The fat cells start to blow up and get bigger like a hamster with food in its mouth. The hamster will release food into his little house as he used his cheeks as a shopping bag, but your fat cells will refuse to release anything and keep the fat cells as full as possible, making them bigger.

The body, skin and hair start to look very unhealthy. Your joints are covered in a connective tissue, and your body needs fat and calcium to maintain the tissue. It's the same as oil in your car. If it's not there, it will stop working and you are in danger of osteoporosis (reduced bone density due to lack of calcium; many low-fat products have no calcium).

Insulin response in the body

Some people are more sensitive, and some people less. Every time you put something into your mouth, you will get an insulin response. Have you seen a heart rate monitor? It goes up. It gives a spike. Insulin does the same in your body.

Imagine you are in the bath, and you are checking those fit men on your phone, and your husband walks in a few times. It's a bit stressful, isn't it? Well, every time you have something to eat or drink, your body has either a small shock, massive shock or no shock, or is happy. Now when you imagine yourself having this shock a couple of times a day .... how do you feel?

Exhausted, don't you?

If your body gets a couple of shocks like this during the day, your metabolism gets exhausted and starts to slow down more than it should.

What kind of food gives your body a shock?

Heavily processed food, with chemicals added to the food. And all the additives that are difficult for your body to recognize as food. Your body is designed to process food. It can digest heavily processed food but with difficulty and at a slower pace. The same with additives.

The good news is that if you eat more of the good food than bad, your body can deal with it. Later, I will provide an example of a week of clean eating to make it more understandable. We are humans, and most of us don't have the capacity and strength to be always good or strict, and we occasionally need chocolate, alcohol, pizza and some small pleasures.

Fat cells + Insulin response + Metabolism = better results, nice body, healthier soul.

Insulin and metabolism

Insulin is a hormone that plays a key role in the body's metabolism and regulates how the body stores and uses glucose and fat. Many cells in the body rely on insulin for energy functions. Insulin has a profound effect on protein, mineral metabolism, carbohydrates and lipids.

The toxic relationship you might create by dieting and bad eating patterns

Have you ever been gaslighted in a relationship?

I know you are wondering what gaslighting is. Let me explain a little.

It's psychological manipulation where a person begins doubting their own sanity. It's very nasty abuse, and it leaves people in a mess. Whoever has been through it knows how horrible it can be. And what it can do to your brain and you as a person. After a gaslighting relationship, I can guarantee you that you will experience some mental health issues.

Let's say that we do this similar crazy abuse to our body and metabolism with food. We give it food, we don't give it (real) food.

We overeat, so the body gets a shock, and then we don't eat at all. We give our body some artificial food or shakes, and then suddenly the body gets clean food again, as we simply need to eat something *normal* to keep sane, and feel better.

This abusive relationship with your body will cause damage to the normal functioning of your body, just as gaslighting will cause damage to your normal emotional functioning.

Then give your body further abuse ...

So much sugar or alcohol that your body is in shock, and is nearly crying and begging us to be nice just for a little while. Then we feel guilty, and for some time, we are good to our body, and then the cycle of abuse starts all over again.

More or less abuse depending on what emotional state we are in. But we can be brutal as it's our body. This is my body, I am going to deal with it, and it's my problem. My body, and that's it.

So, let's think about it. If you have been in an abusive relationship or if you have been gaslighted, you know that recovery takes time. If you have been gaslighted you very possibly are going to need a psychologist for a sanity check.

Recovery takes time.

Some people take longer and others a bit less. Usually, this depends on how long it's been happening and what the damage is. And the same thing is happening to your metabolism and to your body.

Many people start to exercise or eat well, diet or whatever they choose to. But the fact is if you have been harmful to your body and suddenly you are good, your body is a bit slow and is in recovery mode.

The body is not going to respond as quickly as you think or hope. But as I said, everyone is different.

What it means is that sometimes it can take up **to 6 weeks** to see any changes.

Sometimes even during those times, you might gain a kilo up or down and then up again, but because people don't know this after around two weeks of jumping on the scales, they think that "this doesn't work" and give up on what they were doing.

Sometimes we recommend to people not to weigh themselves for 6 weeks, and when they make changes just to pay attention to how they feel.

The number on the scales will change, but your frustration and lack of patience can go through the roof, so there is no need to abuse yourself like this. Just be patient.

People need to understand what's happening and how their bodies works, but as we are humans, most of us are very impatient and we want everything now.

Summary

- If you have been on a rollercoaster ride with diets and starving your body, your metabolism might be on strike or giving you the silent treatment and will not communicate with you. Give it time, it's here for you. You exhausted it. You can only blame yourself, so now work on your patience. It will work again.

- It might take up to 6 weeks for your metabolism to return to work, as it depends on how upset your metabolism is with you or how sensitive your body is to insulin response.

- For 6 weeks, pay attention to your body and how you feel and what your body is craving.

- If you give your metabolism lots of hard work which it can't handle, it won't be happy with you, and it's going to slow down rapidly. And it slows down with age as well.

- If you don't give your fat cells fat, your fat cells will be convinced you are trying to kill them, and will be holding any fat that is coming like mad. And definitely will not send any fat away! You need fat, as it keeps you alive.

- If your insulin has a shock a couple of times a day, it will be knackered and not happy with you. The metabolism and the body will get tired and will slow down.

- Remember, sugar and white flour are powerful mood-altering chemicals. They are there to keep us artificially happy.

- Your body and soul are connected. Just because you don't see the soul, it does not mean it doesn't need to be looked after.

And *mindful eating* is a great pleaser for your soul. I believe we should become soul pleasers when it comes to food, body and mind. But in a healthy way. Without additives, as it's an artificial feeling and it's not real.

What is mindful eating?

Remember when I mentioned Hemingway at the beginning? In simple terms, I would say it is mindful eating. Simply the joy of experiencing the smell, taste, how your body feels. Switching your mind off and focusing on the food that you are eating. Turn your phone or TV off and just enjoy it. Eat slowly.

What does it taste like?

Can you describe it as Hemingway did?

FOR THE SOUL...

LOSING MY MIND

GASLIGHT

What is gaslighting? It is psychological abuse and manipulation in which a person or a group covertly puts doubt into a targeted person or a group of people to make them question their reality and sanity. The person or group will doubt their own perception, judgment, memory. The victim is destabilized, delegitimizes their own beliefs, loses self-confidence, trust in their own judgement, emotions, and perception of reality. The victim is belittled and disoriented.

- The Gaslight Effect. Book written by Dr Robin Stern
- The Gaslight Effect: Lights a way out of an all-too-common dark side of relationships.

"Gaslighting can start even after years of a working relationship where a stressful event or traumatic event can trigger gaslighting. If you are stuck in arguments in your relationship and feel occasionally that you doubt your own sanity, memory or feel a need to record conversations, or you keep on re-reading messages to check what was actually said, you might been gaslighted."

- The famous movie called Gaslight from 1944.
- Have you been called crazy, mental, mad? Maybe it's not you. Maybe you have been gaslighted.

People that have been gaslighted feel they are functioning in a fog. They feel they are not functioning properly; not 100%, not even 70%. They start to lose confidence, and they might start to feel that everything they do, or the way they do is wrong.

They might feel like they lost the person they used to be, and this can make them feel anxious. Many who have been gaslighted struggle with anxiety. They might think to themselves and ask if they were being too sensitive. Questioning their own reality, perception, and sanity.

You might feel as if you are not a loving enough partner if in relationship or question whether your response to your partner is enough or appropriate. Walking on eggshells …

Difficulties making decisions and doubting yourself. Looking for approval.

They start losing pleasure in things they used to do, and their activities become something that has no meaning to them anymore.

They can start feeling like they are living in a fog, they might be aware of it or not. A horrible sense of losing themselves, and things become blurry.

Feeling neurotic, hypersensitive or out of control, struggling to realize what is true and what isn't, is very common.

Just imagine if you have been gaslighted for years, what it does to your mental health. Just like the frog. If you don't jump out, things will get worse. Find a qualified person for a sanity check, as remember that whilst your intentions might have been pure, not everyone functions on this level.

In the book Psychopath Free, Jackson MacKenzie talks about when encountering a psychopathic evil personality, you will possibly feel that you are the "CRAZY" one and might end up acting out of character. It is possible to lose trust and suffer from anxiety just being around people.

If you acted out of character

You might feel ashamed about your behaviour as you might have snapped, but all you did is decided to save yourself. Any emotionally healthy human being is going to react strongly to emotional abuse. As you will be getting closer to the edge, and as this abuse can be extremely hideous and dangerous, remember our self-preservation instinct is one of the strongest instincts we have.

If you end up talking to your friends and family, whilst they have good intentions, they may tell you to ignore people or just smile. But this will make you feel worse, as this abuse is designed to make you think that you are too sensitive or crazy.

I would say it's a "mind F...k"

And if you talk to people that have been through it, you will see the anxious look on their face. Sometimes talking to people is the best thing we can do and sometimes the worst. If you are lucky enough and you speak to someone who has either been through it, or has a knowledge of psychology, they will be able to point you in the right direction. They might say you are being gaslighted, and as you look at what gaslighting is, you might realize its reality. But it's hard without the knowledge.

If you read many self-help or psychology books, you might notice that many writers talk about narcissistic personality disorder and gaslighting. Usually it's a narcissistic game.

When they start to read books on these topics, some people get emotional and simply can't read it, as it triggers the emotions that nearly drove them over the edge. The best is to ask a professional for help if the self-help books get you too emotional or it's too much. *But how amazing to know you are not the crazy one.*

The hidden agenda of gaslighting is, in many cases, the gaining of power over others. Mostly it is controlling abusive behaviour. In many cases of abuse, it's about power. When the gas lightening gets worse or happens for a long time, the target starts to second guess their own memories, thoughts, reality and sanity.

No, you are not crazy, and you were never crazy

Once you can label what's happening to you, this label will help you to realize the problem. And remember, problems are here to be solved. And this one has a solution. Imagine that not your body, but your soul got hit by a bus (I would say in this case got hit by the Airbus).

The damage is there just as if you were slowly boiled to death, but at the last minute, someone pulled the plug, and you survived, unlike the frog who didn't realize the need to jump out until it was too late. You might feel like a different person, and you are living with someone you don't know (you) as the psychological damage changed you, and you feel as though you've lost your true self.

So, we have a label and a problem now. You might have lost your trust in people. EMDR therapy can help, as it's not about having to talk to a psychologist or therapist you don't know and might not trust. EMDR allows *your own* brain to process past traumas and helps you regain balance and slowly bring back you the reality of yourself. It can be bad for 2-3 days after the therapy as it depends on how hard the bus ran over you and how your body and brain will react to therapy. But after therapy, your amazing brain will look after you and will bring you slowly back to where you are supposed to be.

There are a large number of books and YouTube videos to help you understand Gaslighting. The old movie Gaslight might show you how people start to change. And how it drives them "crazy."

As I mentioned earlier, Dr Ramani and Les Carter are very well educated on this topic. (In case you are very busy and don't have time to read books, bath time with YouTube video shorts of around 15 minutes is great therapy, and they will show you that you are a normal emotional human being).

No one wishes to be run over by a bus.

If gaslighting happened to you

Positives

After recovery, I don't have to tell you this is going to make you pretty strong. You become more aware as soon as you realize someone is lying to you and trying to manipulate you, and playing psychological games with you.

You will not join the game. Previously you possibly would have and would react. You will react differently, more aware of your reactions and emotions. Your red flags will now be pretty accurate and, from now on, ready to give you warnings! Pay attention to them.

You have survived this abuse. Congratulations. It is a soul killer for many.

You possibly exchange the circle of people around you as you realize that maybe your empathy and good intentions were, in fact, a magnet for many toxic and manipulative people, and you will start looking after yourself by having more genuine people around you. Emotional blackmail won't work with you now (especially if you had EMDR therapy done, I will introduce you to this therapy later).

If you were one of those people that were always helping others more than yourself, even when they did not need your help as such, you will realize this, and you will put yourself first, finally.

The beautiful new you will show you healthy self - love and no more acceptance of abuse. Unless you need another lesson as you did not learn from this one. Be careful, life tends to keep throwing us into hot water and to keep on jumping out might become too exhausting. Don't end up like the frog.

Everyone has a limit.

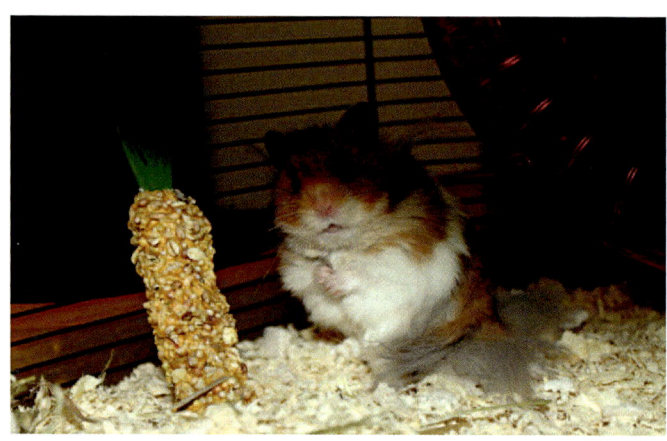

Chapter 4

FAT AND FATTER

SLIM AND SLIMMER & AM I GOING TO DIE?

Lies, sweet little lies

Since you remember, you were never a slim child. When you were a kid, you remember your mum making jokes about not feeding you with milk, but full fat cream, as you looked like you could compete with a baby elephant.

Always had it on your plate. You hate your baby pictures as they remind you more of the hamster Boris with food stuffed in his face, except you had no food there, and most photos were taken just before you had thrown a tantrum because you were hungry.

The school was dreadful as you were always last when it came to running and when there was talk of sports you felt like running but in the opposite direction of where the sport was supposed to happen.

Loose clothes were great, as no one could see how many tyres you were wearing, so you always hoped that you looked like the cool kid with a rather chilled style.

You had been promising for years to yourself that you will sort it out as soon as you are out of school, then out of home, when you change job, or when you change your girlfriend as this one loves junk food and she does not want to eat it alone. Even she doesn't eat for the rest of the day while you do.

You got so tired of those false promises and accepted that the magic number on a scale is not happening, and food makes you happy anyway. And one day, when it gets really bad, you will sort it out.

My first love handles

Hmmmm. My baby photos look ok, except for the crazy ginger hairstyle I had and that I was laughing with my mouth so wide open that I looked like I am finding hysterically funny the fact that Donald Trump is going to be President one day.

Fun days. I got fed, I slept a lot, and when I felt like throwing a tantrum, I did. Happy days.

These days I hardly sleep as the dog is snoring and taking rather a large part of my bed, and the cat is going mental each night on a hunt for my toes. God help me if I move a bit more than I should, as all I get is a crazy attack from my little Siamese tiger. I am so lazy with cooking that I end up eating random food that I find around the house, and when it comes to tantrums, I would love to throw them, but I am too scared I will get locked up in a mental clinic.

When I was a small child, I was so skinny that I was always dreading wearing a skirt, as every time I had it on, my dad told me to bring him the scissors as some threads needed to be cut off, as apparently, the manufacturer had done a bad job. When I brought him the scissors, as I could not see anything, he started to laugh hysterically and apologized, he mistook my legs for threads!

Oh, well, never mind. Yes, my legs were skinny.

My mum used to dread visits to the doctor as she was always told I am underweight and needed to eat more, but for some reason, I was not putting weight on.

If only they knew!

I hated to eat. When I was at school, I used to hide food in my bag and then a week later I somehow remembered it was there, as there was a funny smell coming from my bag, so I used to get rid of it on my way home from school. My mum had no chance to check if I was having anything to eat, as she was leaving to work early, but she always faithfully made me some breakfast.

Poor woman.

I used to skip lunch at school as I found the school food horrible, so sometimes my first meal of the day was in the evening when mum was at home, and she made dinner.

No one ever found out why I was so skinny and was not putting weight on. Even at dinner, I was making a fuss.

When I got older, I thought I am just one of those people that will not put weight on, and I will never have a problem with dieting. Until I had an accident when I was 18, and I was so bored, I binge - watched TV for days and ate everything that I found in the fridge.

To my surprise, I got chubby cheeks like a hamster, and I was out of breath when going up the stairs. I was grumpy, as my body felt heavy, and I had spare tyre I did not like.

That was the first time when I had to lose weight, and I realized how hard it is. And it was taking forever! I was getting on my own nerves by being out of breath all the time and sweating just seeing the stairs.

10 years back, I was happy with my weight until I had a shower and my little nephew Leon walked into the bathroom. He looked over and said, "Auntie Eve, you are fat, what are you going to do about it?". He thought it was hilarious. He started to laugh like crazy and ran off. I looked at my belly and thought, gosh, he is right. What am I going to do about it?

I qualified in personal training and nutrition a year later and shortly afterwards lost my spare tyre …

This happy feeling

You were always the chubby kid. You used to hate your grandma pinching your chubby cheeks and making comments that you should not eat so much, there's too much of you.

You secretly used to go on your bike to the nearest sweet shop with candies, so you could have this fantastic pleasure without listening to any stupid comments.

''Chubby cheek''. You hoped grandma would get fat.

You are an adult now. You are much slimmer than you were as a kid, but you are still surrounded by family that reminds you daily about your rather large days. You exercise daily, and you look ok, but this feeling inside of you that you are not quite good enough is still there. Whenever things go badly, you always buy yourself sweet foods, which makes you feel so nice and good. It's just this happy feeling.

I used to be ok

Maybe you always looked good and never had any problems until you were 15 years old and you started to feel the weight of your body, and you introduced yourself to the crazy roundabouts called diets!

I am sure you see yourself in one of the above, or at least you know someone who this reminded you of. We all remember that terribly skinny kid or a chubby one that hated sports.

When we are kids

When you look a little into your childhood…. some of us were throwing tantrums and were upset as we realized that these two people, mum and dad, are in control, or maybe at least one of them.

Depends on the strength of your parents. A common method of comforting sad children, or emotional children, is offering them food. When you were in distress, your mum or aunt or stressed parent offered you a cake, chocolate, or some other sweet food. Do you remember?

Most parents use this method to comfort upset children, and this becomes a prototype for their later development in chemical dependency. It is attempting to blot out our misery or sadness, and it is a very effective way of quickly forgetting about the problem that made us sad.

The moment you tell kids there is chocolate or sweets, they usually very quickly forget about their tantrum, and their focus changes right away, or very soon after hearing the word chocolate.

Do not blame your parents if you are overweight, as I am sure they tried their best and somehow, they thought or think it's normal, as they were told the same. I am sure many parents are very grateful for chocolate and are well aware that to keep kids quiet or entertained for a while, stick a bag of sweets into their hands.

YOUR BODY TYPE

The 3 scenarios I am talking about are 3 body types.

Your body type is going to have an impact on your ability to achieve whatever you desire to achieve.

Don't use this as an excuse, as there are many examples demonstrating that you can achieve whatever you want in life, as long as you put your mind to it.

There are many examples of celebrities who experience magic weight loss even though their body type is not ideal.

Do not jump to a conclusion of your body type, as most people are a mix of two.

So, let's look at these as guidelines, and I will simplify what it actually means for you.

Ectomorph

Naturally thin body with little body fat or muscle mass

Ectomorph is someone who will get away with eating junk food much easier than many other people, but also someone who is going to struggle to build muscle if they decide to do so.

Higher protein intake should be part of their diet as an ectomorph gaining muscle is harder than for an endomorph.

If you are an ectomorph, running is going to be fairly easy. If you decide to become a bodybuilder be prepared for some hard work. Your body will be a little against you. The thing you have to take on board is you are used to living in a lean body that is possibly quite quick, and you are used to being light.

If you become a bodybuilder, your running will slow down, and running will be much harder work than you are used to. Your heart and cardio are going to have to carry the extra weight of large muscles.

If you eat pizza or junk food a few times a day, you are probably easily getting away with it. But be careful. This will change with age. If you are a young individual, enjoy this. You will have to be a little careful if you don't exercise as your metabolism is going to change.

Earlier for women, around 18 years of age and for men around 24.

Guidelines for an ectomorph on nutrition

This can be misleading as it really depends on your lifestyle. If you are a builder, you can eat more carbs and possibly unhealthy food than a person who works in an office.

Use common sense as you know your body better than any nutritionist or any personal trainer. All it means is if you become a bodybuilder, you will have to work harder at the gym and eat more than mesomorphs.

Remember, you know your body best, and you can feel yourself if you are putting weight on, either muscle or fat. Listen to your body.

Common food guidelines for ectomorphs

Carbohydrates: 60%

Protein: 30%

Fats: 10%

Mesomorph

If you are a mesomorph, I would say you are lucky. Whether you decide to be a bodybuilder or marathon runner, your body will work with you.

As a mesomorph, you tend to be naturally lean and muscular, broad shoulders, narrow waist and hips. Mesomorphs are naturally athletic and tend to be suited to a wide variety of sporting activities.

You have an advantage against the other two body types. Either you decide to do marathon running or become a bodybuilder, it will be easier than for your colleagues who are ectomorphs or endomorphs.

Common food guidelines for mesomorph

Carbohydrates: 50%

Protein: 30%

Fats: 20%

Endomorph

Endomorphs gain fat easier than other body types. This body type is naturally predisposed to the storage of fat. They tend to be apple or pear shaped and carry large amounts of body fat. Endomorphs are predisposed to gain a reasonable degree of muscle mass, even if this is often overlooked due to a predisposition for fat storage.

Endomorphs are physically strong individuals even without using the gym every day.

If you are planning on becoming a marathon runner, be prepared for hard work and eating pretty clean. Everything is possible, but as I mentioned with ectomorph, you are used to living in a strong body, and you might enjoy body building more than running.

Common food guidelines for endomorphs

Carbohydrates: 40%

Protein: 30%

Fats: 30%

The saying I look at pizza, and I gain 2 kgs might be familiar to you. If you want to be lean, you will get away with eating pizza and junk food a little less than other body types.

The cleaner you eat, the better for you.

You should follow guidelines of 80% good and 20% bad food, but it's easy enough once you get rid of the addictions.

Many people are not exclusively one body type, rather a combination of two or more. Individuals with a small frame, little muscle mass and a tendency to store body fat could be considered an ectomorph with endomorphic tendencies.

Understanding your body type will help *you, especially if you compare yourself with others when it comes to dieting and achievements.*

Many people will put themselves into one category, but they might be a different type, but their habits drove them to an unhealthy weight and body shape. Once you change your diet, then you will realize which body type you are. You might only get away with having 2 pizzas a week, while others can have 3-4, but you can always move things around once you have a better understanding.

Keep in mind your lifestyle is probably the main reason why you look the way you look. Genetics plays some role, but what we look like is the biggest indicator of how much knowledge we have, and how much we care about our physical and mental well - being.

Hurdles are there to be to be jumped. Nothing else. Take it as a challenge if your body proposition is a little against you. There have been enough people who have proved already whatever we want, we can achieve. Work out how you are going to do it and do it. Have fun. Looking after your body should become *your hobby and joy.*

There are many ways we can approach weight loss. We can see the body type and create a diet (daily food income).

We can use calorie counting techniques and simply create a deficit, either by food or exercise or ideally using both.

Frequently explaining how the body works along with some simple tricks and clean eating, so there is no hassle with calorie counting.

FOR THE SOUL...

AM I GOING TO DIE?

Panic attacks

Many people have so much stress in their life they forgot about selfcare, as they manage to put everyone else before themselves, they simply overcooked things and moved from anxiety to panic attacks. It can be one of many reasons why people develop panic attacks.

Panic attacks can be very frightening and can come from nowhere and without warning.

It's a sudden and very intense moment of fear, and it triggers physical reactions. When a person is experiencing a panic attack, it can feel as if they are losing control and can't function. They can feel like they are dying or having a heart attack. Shaking, sweating, shortness of breath, hot flashes, nausea, dizziness, faintness, chest pain and many more.

It can be very frightening.

After major <u>stress in life</u>, you might experience panic attacks. Death or serious illness of a loved one, a traumatic event, prolonged sleeplessness, exhaustion, prolonged abuse either mental or physical, bad injury, accident, divorce, newborn baby, prolonged financial problems, can be triggers. If you are sensitive to negative emotions, stress, abuse, you are going to be more prone to panic attacks.

Panic attacks affect more women than men.

Panic attacks can become a big part of one's life and if untreated, it can leave you living in a constant state of fear, and it will feel like they are ruining your life. Panic attacks can cause the development of phobias, avoidance of social situations, increased risk of suicide, depression, anxiety, and other psychiatric problems. Also, problems at school, work or financial problems as your work capacity will decrease. Depression.

<u>Regular exercise plays a role in protecting against anxiety and panic attacks.</u>

Treatment

I will get through this

Finding a qualified therapist. Becoming more aware of what triggers you.

Selfcare such as yoga, breathing exercises, meditation, physical exercise, good eating patterns, better sleeping patterns, better self – care, and all focus more on the positive. Therapy might explain a lot, and by understanding things and knowing what we are dealing with, can be a great help.

Don't forget finding a therapist is a great way to look after your soul. Just as a body needs a doctor, sometimes your mind does too. Just because you cannot see the wound on your soul doesn't mean it's not there and doesn't need treatment. The soul takes much longer to heal than your physical body. That's why even more so we should look after our mental health.

If your body got hit by a bus, the impact would be pretty nasty, and sometimes it's our soul that gets hit, but not the body. Our mind has an amazing tendency to protect us and switches off, but our body tells us something is wrong in the form of anxiety, depression, panic attacks, and many other signs, but we sometimes start treating the body but not the soul.

The soul is trying to tell us something is wrong and uses the body to get our attention.

Look after your soul. It's the only one you have got. It deserves to be treated and looked after.

If you bottle it all up, it is still there. One day a crisis can uncover all the emotional traumas, and you are going to have a lot to deal with, but it might be a blessing as you will finally have to deal with the underlying issues.

Sadness can make you ill.

When you don't feel physically well, it's normal to go for a checkup. The moment we don't feel mentally well, we should go for a sanity check and make sure we check our mind and soul. Nothing is wrong with that, as all of us struggle sometimes.

Well, not as much as psychopaths. Did you know psychopaths don't have the basic 5 emotions we have? They don't suffer with fear, anxiety, lack of empathy, guilt and remorse.

Did you just think to yourself how great it would be not to feel fear, anxiety and not to fall apart sometimes when people are nasty?

I guess it would be great not to feel some of these, but also remember these feelings are sometimes warnings that something is wrong. These feelings are also protecting us as they send us signals we are not ok, and we need fixing and healing.

The body is a soul's house.

1 in 6 people are a danger to our mental health. It means we are in a shark's pool. We get warnings about what is healthy or unhealthy for our body all the time, but no one warns us about what is unhealthy for our souls.

Many people start recovery after their breakdowns and burnouts, but frankly if they had had knowledge beforehand and learnt to protect their soul just as much as their body, they would not have experienced so many mental health problems.

Sometimes we grow up in toxic families that were very unhealthy for our mental health, or sometimes we end up in very toxic relationships, and we refuse to do anything about it, and we stay in those situations for too long. It can then become normal for us, as we forget what it's like to be loved in a healthy way.

Then toxic becomes normal, even if it's slowly killing the soul.

Many times, we know there is something wrong, but we choose to ignore it.

Before we know it, we can end up like the frog in boiling water, losing the ability to jump out.

I am not saying to leave (sometimes I would say RUN), but psychologist, couples' therapy and books are such a great help to gain the knowledge we need to understand what we are dealing with, what the outcomes are, and why we react the way we do.

Someone has already been through it and found a solution to many things, so we don't need to. The books and therapists are very well informed and have seen most, if not all, before.

I understand we are all busy, but even on your way to work, instead of listening to music, you can listen to audio books about the problem you seek to sort out. You are not the first one with the problem you have, and there is a very good chance someone has worked the problem out.

You will be amazed at how accurate some books are, and you might end up on an emotional roller-coaster of being both angry and happy that you hear this. You might get angry, as you will realize it's a very common thing, but no one told you before, and most people were telling you it's normal, grow up, suck it up, or something similar.

You might find out that you are boiling in your skin, but there is an answer to nearly everything, as many psychologists already had seen it before. Your empathy can kill you if you use it for the wrong people. Be careful. Your responsibility is to look after that person you are looking at every morning in the mirror. Learn to take care of your soul.

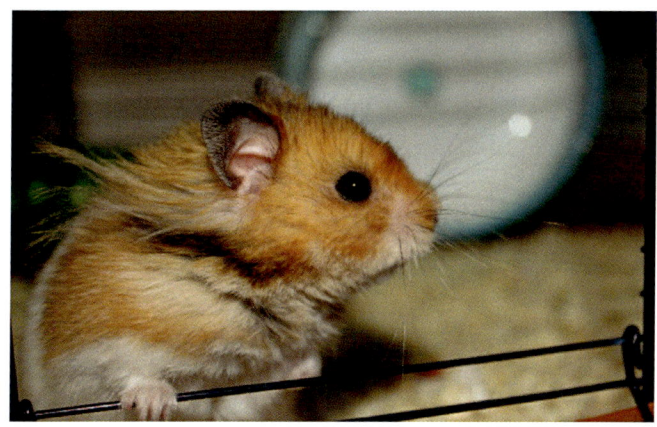

Chapter 5

SLOW IS STEADY, STEADY IS FAST & FIRING FIELD

Jolene and numbers

Numbers! Numbers are everywhere! Jolene works in sales and uses numbers all the time. Numbers work! Of course, they work. She knows that.

She has been trying to lose weight for some time, but no luck and suddenly she realizes that she has been eating too many calories! That must be it! She's finally worked it out.

She goes a little crazy, and she sees numbers everywhere! She goes to the shop where everyone is yelling at each other as they can't hear each other over the face masks, but all she can see and hear are numbers!

She gets home, and whilst feeding her hamster, she tries to work out how many calories Boris is eating daily, as he is still rather huge, even after his daily marathons. "I must reduce his calories too," she thinks to herself. Boris looks rather terrified looking at her but still happily runs around. She even starts to count how many rounds he does while she is having the revelation of why she cannot lose any weight.

She is feeling like an idiot, as it was so obvious. She thinks of the number on the scale.

All she can think of is numbers.

She gets excited as she feels now she knows where she is going wrong, and she can fix this. She is becoming a little obsessed with this, but it doesn't matter as long as she will get to where she has been trying to for a very long time.

She goes to the shop and starts turning the bags of her favourite food around to read the nutrition labels and starts counting how many calories are inside them.

Let's have a look at the guidelines if we do use calorie counting and the common mistakes.

How do we calculate and use calorie burn in weight loss?

The calculation of your calories burned daily

For an accurate calculation, we use the Harris Benedict formula. To determinate your basal metabolic rate (BMR), you can do a simple calculation using these guidelines. This is a more accurate calculation than using your bodyweight alone.

For underweight people, this calculation will underestimate caloric needs. For extremely overweight people, it will over estimate calorie needs, as this calculation does not consider the amount of lean body mass.

You can of course, use the internet and simply put the numbers in an online calculator. Just search for BMR calculation.

WOMEN BMR;

655+ (9.6 times weight in kg) + (1.8times height in cm) - (4.7 times age) =

MEN BMR:

66+ (13.7 times weight in kg) + (5 times height in cm) - (6.8 times age) =

<u>Example of female 38 years old 172cm high and 58 kg weight</u>

655 + (9.6 times 58 = 556.8) + (1.8 times 172= 309.6) - (4.7times 38= 178.6) = 1342.8 calories a day and she goes to the gym 2-3 times a week.

Now you have to multiply by activity: Total Daily Energy Expenditure (TDEE)

Sedentary   BMR times 1.2 (little or no exercise, desk job)

Lightly active BMR times 1.375 (little exercise/sports 1-3 times days /week)

Mod activity   BMR times 1.55 (moderate exercise/sports 3-5 days /week)

Very active   BMR times 1.725 (hard exercise/ sports 6-7 days/week)

Extra active   BMR times 1.9 (hard daily exercise/sports and physical jobs)

So, your BMR is 1342.8cal and you do little activity.   1342.8 times 1.375 = **1846.35 calories.**

This number gives you your (TDEE) **Total Daily Energy Expenditure.**

You can do a workout and burn 250 calories and have one snack less, giving a further saving of 250 calories. Be careful, though, as psychologically you are going to think that after exercise you must eat. Of course, you will eat, but remember you need a calorie deficit, so going to the gym does not mean you can eat like an elephant the moment you get home.

When people start losing weight, many get a little hungry and feel panic as part of them is leaving. They are losing body fat, and hate their body fat, but they also feel a bit strange to start losing it. They start to overthink the process, asking whether it's healthy. They feel a little weird as it's part of their body, and it was with them for a decade, so the thought of a new body can be a little odd and scary.

Don't worry, it's normal to have these thoughts. Your body fat was giving you an emotional rollercoaster, you might be a little addicted to it. You might be addicted to the crazy diet roundabout and constantly trying to lose weight, so the moment it happens, it can be emotional for some people. Suddenly the ups and downs won't be there, as it's finally happening. You might have to study your own feelings and brain and ask why you are feeling the way you are.

Ask yourself why and what makes you go up and down. Some people will have a great boost as they see it happening, but the next minute they're feeling down and sceptical as they are scared they will fail, or it's going to stop, and they will not make their goal again. Just breathe.

Not everyone can handle the change. Sometimes you need time to adapt to it.

People often ask why someone burns 1800cal and someone else 2300cal. You can see a difference between a female, for example, of 55kgs and a female of 85kgs. The body of an 85kg female has a much harder job to carry a body of 85kg from A to B than a 55kg body, as it's simply heavier. The female of 85kg is going to have a larger number of calories used than the 55kg female, as the workload for the body is much bigger. A lorry is going to use more fuel than a small car.

TDEE is your total daily calories burned by your body. We use this as a guideline to work out a deficit.

Note: Many people who are a little OCD (obsessive compulsive disorder) find counting calories good, as they usually have good control and they follow routines strictly.

What should be your daily deficit and the best way and why

1) Remember how clever your body is? Your body looks after you, so you cannot go crazy with it.

2) Your body has memorized the weight you are and takes it into account, and tries to keep it there. If you start with a crazy fast diet, your body will simply not let you, as it looks after you, so it's going to drive your metabolism down to a minimum or will give you crazy cravings to make you eat.

3) If you want to create a healthy deficit for the body without driving yourself crazy with an emotional roller-coaster, where your body creates massive cravings as it's thinking you are trying to starve it and kill it, your daily deficit **should be:**

250cal deficit in food daily and **250cal** deficit daily in exercise.

This will create a deficit of 500 cal a day which comes to **3500cal a week.**

3500cal = 0.9lb (0.41kg) = comes to 182000 calories a year = 21kg of fat weight loss without a risk of the Yo-Yo effect.

4) Research shows if you do it slowly, without putting your body into panic mode your body will burn more fat and keep you lean. If you go with a bigger deficit than this, research shows that body fat is more likely to return and usually more than before. The Yo-Yo effect.

5) Your body works for you and is trying to keep you alive. Be clever and lose weight slowly, and your body will not panic, and you have less chance you are going to have an emotional roller

coaster with emotional eating, as your hormones will be under control.

6) It's better to go slowly and healthily as it's going to stay off rather than return to the original. Remember, if you eat healthily, it's coming to a total of 182,000 cal a year, and that is 22 kg of fat lost in a year! This is the magic weight loss that celebrities do. I am sure you have noticed they hire a personal trainer, the knowledge is there.

7) Slow is steady, steady is fast.

8) Let's say that you had a really bad, day and you ate much more than you were supposed to. Well, don't panic, that's fine. The next day create a little bigger deficit to compensate. BUT try to stick to your daily calories going forward. Let's say the next day, you push it a little higher and go for a run and eat the same calories, or if you have no time, you simply cut your daily calorie allowance. The run would be much better as cardio exercise will speed up your metabolism for another 24 hours, and let me also remind you how great you feel after workout.

9) If you failed a day, do not feel emotional about it, you are only human, and we all do it. Even personal trainers. But try not to do it every day! If it happens twice a week, it's ok, but be careful as you don't want to have a crazy rollercoaster, as your body might go into panic mode.

10) Remember, if you are a female, don't expect a 0.5 kg a loss a week just before your period. Most women will be slightly higher or still the same weight, as the body is holding fluids.

11) Don't worry about it, as if you stick to it the following week, your weight will go down again and possibly even more. If you are having crazy sugar cravings, use the chocolate technique, I described earlier.

12) At around 4 weeks, the weight loss can stop. But it can also be after 2 weeks or more. It depends, but it's going to happen a few times during your weight loss. Just ignore it. Sometimes it varies even if you do everything right. As I mentioned before, your body memorizes your body weight, and after a few weeks, it's thinking something is wrong, as you are losing weight. As it's not sure what is happening, your body needs to have a think about it, and check if everything is functioning well, as your body is getting smaller, it's going to desperately hold the weight for a couple of days, or even perhaps two weeks before it allows you to lose some more.

13) After you have lost some weight, remember to redo the calculation again, as your body is lighter. Your daily calorie deficit will be smaller. If you keep using the initial value, you will plateau. Once you lost approximately 5kgs, you will need a further reduction of 100 calories. Your stomach is getting a little smaller as well, don't worry that you are going to be 'missing' food, it won't. It's adjustment to a change.

14) It's simple, don't overthink it. Remember, your body is trying very hard to keep you alive, its only job on top of taking you from A to B. Look after it, and learn to understand why your body functions the way it does, as having the *knowledge* it will not give you an emotional rollercoaster.

15) Many people get upset when they realize that their weight isn't decreasing anymore, and start eating a lot again and it all goes to waste. Then they try to go back to it and start to experience the yo-yo effect.

16) There is one other thing to mention as well. About calories and labels. They are 20% + or – in accuracy. Whilst the food labels and calculations are not very accurate, they are accurate enough for what you need.

17) Remember if you do it like this you, will not regain the weight in 5 years' as most people do, as it gives you time to adapt to the changes and adopt a new lifestyle. And your body will not go crazy with cravings. It's healthier to go slowly. It will be easier for your brain to adjust to the changes.

Few more facts for you

If you eat more often and smaller portions, your metabolism will keep working without going to <u>sleep</u> (when people starve themselves, the metabolism goes into sleep mode as there is simply no work) or panic mode when concerned about starvation (on both occasions, it works at minimum).

Insulin in your body drives glucose in your blood into cells of the body for its use. It sends glucose to the liver and muscles, where its stored as glycogen. Glucose will be driven to other cells through the body. High glycogenic foods and refined carbohydrates (heavily processed food) tend to cause insulin levels to spike (as I mentioned earlier, you just freaked it out too many times, and its stopped working), and it favours fat storage and suppresses fat burning as a fuel. Spiking often results in a subsequent crash in blood glucose and creates tiredness, hunger and possibly overeating.

We want to avoid insulin resistance as much as possible, as it's associated with increased body fat and tiredness during the day. Aerobic exercise has a positive effect on reducing insulin resistance by increasing insulin sensitivity, especially within the muscle tissue.

Go for a run.

It's great for your skin, your mental health, and you are going to sleep well and feel great. Even if you go for a run twice a week. A little is more than nothing. Maybe it's going to be your little escape from the crazy roundabout at home or work. You might notice after exercise a boost in your ability to deal with stress.

Remember, one man's food is another man's poison. People from around the world have different diets, different macronutrients and still manage to be healthy.

We can tell people that some foods are better, but we have no intention of changing things too much for people, as they simply love their own food and culture.

Each body is different, and paying attention to how you feel is more important in the long term, so long as it's positive and you are not lying to yourself.

As I mentioned earlier about addictions, we feel satisfied the moment we eat food as we have satisfied the cravings. But how you feel half an hour after is a different story. And that's where we pay attention to how your body responds to food. 30 minutes after consumption, you will be feeling energetic or sleepy, and the same for your brain. Pay attention to how you feel immediately after eating and half an hour after eating. How do your body and mind feel?

Calorie counting works if you do it correctly. Try not to drive yourself crazy with it.

Mostly emotions are stronger than your body.

If your mind is there, your body will follow.

That's why I want you to become more aware of how food makes you and your body feel in the long term. In the short term, we do have addictions, and we already know how well they work.

Possibly you can see that you can easily fit a couple of Snickers bars into your daily calorie count, that's why it's nonsense when people think that fitness people never eat chocolate. The reason fitness people don't eat as much unhealthy food, is that we gained the knowledge and learnt to look after our bodies and became aware of how we feel.

It becomes a habit to eat well, just as it was a habit to eat bad food. It becomes a joy as you are simply happy in your body, so your health becomes more important to you. You learn how to get rid of the addictions slowly, so your body doesn't send you crazy signals to give me some chocolate, or I will go crazy, on a daily basis.

Have you noticed that when you eat a chocolate bar the next day, your body sends you cravings to eat the same chocolate bar again? Or some other addictive food?

If you calorie count, there are many apps for you to use to assist you. If you want to be slim, eat well and if you want to be slim and look good exercise as well.

FOR THE SOUL...

FIRING FIELD

100 billion neurons

What am I talking about here? Your brain. Give or take a few billion. And yes, they do fire on average about 200 times per second at a speed of 150 miles per second.

The brain is a network of cells and neurons that use electrical and chemical signals to communicate. You are an electrical and chemical field. And chemicals drive you.

Your brain records everything and every experience has an emotion that is stored in your body.

What happens to your computer if you keep throwing viruses at it or if there are simply too many viruses detected on your computer? It starts to slow down and break unless you get rid of the virus. If you have permanent stress, emotional, financial or any other stress, for a long time, you feel sad, frustrated, exhausted most of the time. What do you think is happening in your electrical and chemical field, how do you think your computer will function after a while?

Your neurons are firing, and you can create an addiction to negative emotions, stress, sadness. Your sympathetic nervous system is activating a fight or flight response. The rush of adrenalin creates an emotional state of being, which can create an addiction to negative emotions as the release of adrenalin is a strong emotional response.

Your thinking, your emotions, your state of being, has an effect on your electrical and chemical state. Living in stress, sadness or any other negative emotional or physical state you are living in survival mode. And survival mode can become your new normal as you get used to it. Do not accept it.

When your sympathetic nervous system is on high alert or becomes overactive due to stress, the body's response can lead to PTSD, depression, anxiety, panic attacks or physical illness. People who have been under prolonged emotional, physical or mental stress usually develop one of these symptoms. The longer you are under stress in survival mode, the bigger the chance of developing psychological problems.

There is a problem for many people who get used to stress, or who are addicted to stress or grew up in very emotional, unstable families or environments where some of them were used as an emotional punch bag by their parents, or were under constant stress from the high demands of their families. These people in many cases, never realized they were permanently stressed, and stress is their 'normal'. Usually, it is just a question of time before something happens, and these people suffer a breakdown. The box has got filled up, and they can't put anything in it anymore, but someone will try to squeeze a little more in. Many have lived in survival mode their whole lives, without realizing it.

Many people like this are looking for stressful jobs and stressful environments as it's their 'home'. Their childhood was stressful, adulthood is as well and so much strength is needed not to suffer from health issues when you think about it.

Many people when young became carers for their families or parents and they learnt to put their own needs second, which usually stays with them for life. It's again their 'unhealthy normal'. But as many of us are missing the knowledge, we 'feel' that something is not right, but we struggle to work out what it is, as we were never told any different.

When we do something enjoyable, our brain rewards us with good feelings. This comes from eating, pleasurable drugs, activities that we enjoy, exercising. As it feels good, our brain is telling us to repeat the behaviour, so we get rewarded. The problem happens when the 'pleasure' is in fact, unhealthy. Imagine if you have lots of stress and you find something that gives you 'pleasure' feelings. How easy it is to become addicted to something if you are under high stress or lived in high stress for a long time.

Have a look at the scans of a normal brain and a stressed brain.

If you have unhealthy patterns or behaviours, it's very important to have a look where they come from and why you created them. Maybe they were your survival mechanism for a long time, but they might cause you lots of problems in adult life.

If you are surrounded by mentally unhealthy individuals for prolong time, you are very likely to develop mental health problems.

Appetite for destruction

Addiction is a brain disease. And you can be addicted to nearly anything.

What are your addictions?

Most of us are addicted to certain foods since a young age. We usually develop very similar or the same addictions as our parents.

Around 70% of obese people learnt their food addictions and food habits from their parents. Most people like to blame their obesity on DNA and tell you that their parents were never slim, or it runs in the family. I am sorry. But I disagree, and I will say that a bigger problem is unhealthy behaviour patterns from the family, and DNA is mostly just an excuse to avoid changing habits.

Most people are born without anxiety and mental health problems. They are born with a healthy brain scan. As they grow up in chaos, they can learn destructive behaviours from their parents and consequently develop the same mental health problems as their parents. DNA plays a role, but have a think about it. You were born with a healthy brain. How is stress affecting you, and have you noticed when you are under a huge amount of stress, you copy one of your parent's behaviors? Which one? And what health issues this parent have?

I changed my habits after I qualified in nutrition and learnt to like myself and take care of myself better. Before then, my habits were horrendous. After I learnt how the food industry functions and how they are benefiting from my unhealthy lifestyle, I felt like an idiot, and I felt embarrassed at how well they had played me. These days I am in charge and you will be too.

The moment you have sugar, msg, or many other addictive stuffs, the chemical reaction in your brain sends a signal of pleasure, and within hours your brain is craving the same 'feeling'. Within hours your brain sends you to the fridge or a cupboard to get the chocolate out, as it's simply craving the sugar or the chemicals in the product which gave you the 'good feeling'. Of course, it can also be alcohol or something else. It's very simply explained, but possibly you can also guess why it is nearly impossible to maintain a 'diet'.

Have you noticed the unhealthier food you eat, the more you are craving it? Do you have a habit of passing a petrol station or a takeaway, and you feel a desire to stop and get a snack, and you are struggling not to? The moment you are pass the place or the shop, your taste cells and brain become more active and send you the signal of "I want to feel good".

The more you are getting, the more your brain is firing and creating a chemical imbalance, and you are becoming addicted. The same happens in unhealthy relationships. The adrenalin rush you are getting from unhealthy people, or unhealthy places is a very strong emotional footprint on your soul. There is more complex stuff on relationships and the patterns we have, and I would recommend people to find a therapist to have a look more deeply into the problem. Still, I want you to be aware, how easy it is to create an addiction to unhealthy food and unhealthy life style.

I would like to mention that until you realize that the reason you are making changes is purely for your good, it will be nearly impossible to change your habits.

You can have many relationships in life and many houses and cars. But you are only going to have one body and one mind.

We might be going to have to re-wire the brain to healthy homeostasis, but without knowing what is happening, it is difficult.

You need to start rewiring your brain into, "I am going to look after this body, I have only got this one".

How do you re-wire it? The first step is to realize you are not in a healthy state of being. Start asking, "when was the last time you felt 'good' or 'normal'?". What happened that created an imbalance? Psychologists usually look at your childhood as it's very common to create unhealthy survival habits that can kill you later on in life or make you ill. Being your own psychologist sometimes can help if you are a very self-aware person, but sometimes we all need help to be pointed in the correct direction.

Many people where one or both parents were alcoholic, or simply suffered from abandonment or an abusive relationship, often struggle with self-valuation and create bad coping patterns that are self-destructive in terms of never feeling that they are good enough. They were never valued and loved the way they deserved to be as children, and their patterns can easily lead them towards abusive relationships, as they have a deep belief they don't deserve to be loved, whereas that's what they crave. They are often people that can love deeply, and they get hurt badly as many people will take their love and care for granted. Lack of their own self-care and self-valuation can be destructive, and it's important to heal and sort out the problem. Often if they don't heal, they are prone to addictions and addictive behaviour.

Find a photo of yourself when you were a child and have a look at this child. What would you say to this child? Imagine it's the child you love the most. Is this what you wanted for this child? What advice would you tell this child with the biggest love you can feel? Would you be happy for the life this child has? Or would you say, look after yourself, take care of yourself and leave some people and some relationships…? Make changes, change the job and your patterns? Love yourself more? What would it be? Go and find a photo of yourself.

Addiction is a nasty chemical that tells you – you need me to survive. It's a nasty relationship where you believe you won't survive without the abuser, who occasionally seems nice and helpful. High and low and hot and cold can be addictive.

Exercise for you: When you are brushing your teeth in the morning, have a look at the person in the mirror and ask yourself, how do I treat this human being? Do I let this person get bullied? Do I look after this person's mental health? Do I respect this person? How do I look after this person's body? Do I give it good food? If this person in the mirror was my loved child, would I be happy with how I treat this kid? The small child is still inside.

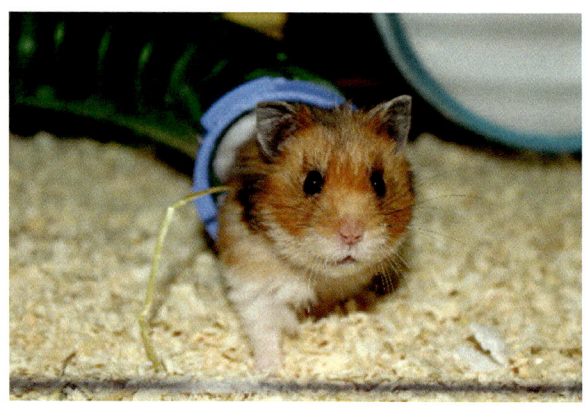

Chapter 6

VEGANS, GAME CHANGERS, EMPATHS AND BUDDHA & ALL THAT YOU HAVE IS YOUR SOUL

Do you not feel crazy sometimes as there is always some new research and one moment everything is healthy, and next year it's apparently killing you? Should I eat this, or should I not? Should I eat eggs, or maybe not? Should I eat processed food, should I not? What should I eat?

Should I eat at all?

Jolene is Googling whether vegetarians or vegans are slim, as she literally doesn't know what to eat anymore. Boris is driving her up the wall, as she has not made it to the gym for the last two weeks, and Mr. Boris looks like he is training for the Olympic Games.

She trains to have a small butt, but apparently, it is fashionable to have one the size of a horse (not a racehorse) these days. She wonders if she should keep her gym membership active, or save money and get herself some butt implants.

She starts to wonder what it's like to sit on one of those. They might even keep her warm? Is it comfy? Might get them for the winter, she thinks to herself.

Stop the craziness

Should you go and meditate, or should you go and do some karate? Should you try to get a supermodel body or not, as lately they promote a larger size than those athletic gazelles that everyone once admired?

What is right and what is wrong?

You even wonder to yourself if you should get a girlfriend, even though you have been dating men the whole of your life. You've always thought women were gorgeous. Maybe I should?

Should I get those diet pills? Maybe they will put me out of this misery, or perhaps they will put me in hospital?

Sometimes there is so much advice around, and so much we should do or not do, or follow or unfollow.

We forget to do things that are good for our souls. We follow something that is supposed to be good. We are not even sure if it is good, but someone said … so we go for it. Sometimes it's more like torture, but we still do it as it's apparently supposed to be good.

Does it feel good?

Some people follow something as they are lonely and need to be part of something. Being part of a group gives people a feeling of importance, also being a part of a group gives people a false sense of safety. To be part of something provides feelings of higher self-worth, self-esteem, status and some sort of identity. Some people need it, and it makes them feel good. Yes, we are back to feelings and how we value ourselves or how we want others to value us.

Some people are not sure, and being part of a larger group gives them a secure feeling, as surely so many people can't be wrong. Many people have really good reasons why they follow something, and many have no idea. What about yourself? Can you answer for yourself?

Do whatever makes sense to you and makes you happy, but always be true to yourself. For mental well-being and spiritual growth, you must develop your own religion and beliefs and not blindly adopt your parents or someone else. If you want to be happy, be true to yourself. If you want to be slim and happy, you need to develop healthy self love towards your body and start working on your relationship with your own body. Take care of it … it's the only one you have got.

I have met people who followed all the healthy guidelines and became terminally ill at the age of 50. I have met people who smoked and drank most of their adult life and died at the age of 80. Whatever you choose when it comes to food, it is totally up to you, as long as you are paying attention to how your body and soul feel. It's your life and your choice. Your responsibility.

Many people get married as they are fighting loneliness, or looking for a (false) sense of security that marriage is supposed to provide. It kills loneliness, keeps them busy, but marriage is hard work. You will be busy and let's hope it's going to go well and you will be happy. If not, you will be happily divorced a few years later. And you will join the group of single ones. Have you noticed how many people gain weight as soon as they get married? Is it laziness, comfort, or simply no longer trying to look after themselves as someone 'loves them' so they don't need to look nice anymore?

To keep you relaxed, most people say that their second marriages are happier. There is hope for everyone. We learn from our mistakes, at least we hope we do.

Marriage can be heaven or hell. Let's hope for heaven.

People's choices and reasons when it comes to food

Vegetarians

- Vegetarians are concerned about killing animals. They are happy to eat the products of animals, like eggs, milk, dairy, as you don't kill the animal to get it.
- For many people, it is also a spiritual concern, as they feel it is ethically not right to kill an animal. They also feel that not killing and consuming animals can raise their spiritual vibration. Reducing animal suffering means their karma is improving. For many people, it was and is about spiritual

growth. Many people are animal lovers and feel it's wrong for them to be part of the killing of any living soul.

Vegans

- When it comes to veganism, there are three main reasons. One is environmental, as animals are very inefficient food producers. Instead of growing tons of plants to feed an animal and eating the animal, it's better just to eat the plants.
- Secondly, ethical reasons for not killing animals.
- Lastly, concerns about health. When you think about it, no research tells you vegetables and fruits are making you ill. No research tells you that eating fruit or vegetables is bad for you or gives you cancer or any illnesses, or has a negative impact on you. Of course, there are some intolerances and peanut allergies, but that's a different story. Many people believe that having a diet based on fruit and vegetables is a much healthier diet.
- For many, it comes to one or all of health, environment and reducing suffering.

Game Changers

- I recommend you watch the film Game Changers. I don't want to talk about it as much here, as having to watch it will give you a better idea. I like it very much, but I know many who don't like it and doubt it, make your own mind up. It's a documentary on how people who only eat plant products feel and the effects of exercise if you do not eat meat products.
- Another couple of film recommendations: That Sugar Film, Globesity.
- Your own path in life and your religion. You need your own views to be happy, whatever *is closest to your soul.*

Empath's and sensitive people

- There is also a group of people called empaths. These people have sensitive souls and are very sensitive to energies and vibrations. Some empaths don't eat meat as they say they feel the anxiety of the animals just before they were killed. Some empaths feel a very close connection to animals, and feel they cannot eat them.
- Some empaths and sensitive people can have addictions.
- People with high sensitivity to energies can become overweight, as extra padding can provide protection from negative energies.
- They can overeat to cope with difficult people or emotional stress.

- For empaths or sensitive people, food can became a plaster or a medicine. Which can make them unhealthy and further it's a short - term fix.

- Most common addiction is sugar and carbohydrates (not only for sensitive people).

- I know many clients (and me personally) that after eating food with MSG get headaches. The more you can get rid of additives in food, the more sensitive you will become as well, as your body is starting to come out of a toxic state and be healthier. It's the same, as if you have no alcohol for a while, you will feel and get drunk more quickly.

Some common questions you can ask yourself

- When you are emotionally overwhelmed or stressed, do you overeat?

- Do you feel less protected from stress and toxicity when you are thin?

- Do you get mood swings from sugar, caffeine, junk food? Are you aware of it?

- If you answer yes, you are probably aware of how food makes you feel in the longer term.

- Are you using food, drinks, sugar to help you cope with stress?

Common sense

Use common sense when you think about food. Everything that nature is giving us without too much human input never made anyone ill or sick or gave them imbalances that can cause depression and mood swings and physical illness.

Nearly everything that humans have modified is unhealthy for the body and mind. Some things less, and some more.

Research shows that many additives and drugs used in the food industry negatively impact our brain. In Britain, every second person will get cancer in their lifetime. I understand we get old and our body is tired, but it might be ok to get cancer when we are 70 or 80 rather than at 30?

We get consumed in this material world, and we try to be healthy so much that we have foods that are great and healthy for us just outside the kitchen window in our gardens. But we go to a shop and buy stuff that is supposed to keep us young forever and has been created in a factory where the product never sees daylight. We get into such a mind fog that we are looking for good and healthy stuff in the wrong places, and we start to lose common sense, or we make excuses and go for processed food as it requires less preparation and cooking time.

Some studies clearly show processed carbohydrates are making us ill. I do agree to some extent, and I don't like to tell people to never eat them. I love my local pizza, and there is nothing wrong with having a lovely pizza and glass of wine occasionally.

Of course, you can stop and make massive changes, but psychologically those changes don't last as we are humans. And instead of sorting out things, we need to have a think what changes we need to make to have more positive emotions in life. The moment many of us get frustrated, we go for sugar, food, carbs and alcohol. It's our weakness as human beings.

I recommend trying a week of clean eating just to bring awareness to *feelings* when it comes to food and how it makes you feel. From then on, you will change your relationship with food. You don't know how good you can feel until you have tried it. You have been living in this heavily numbed, drugged state from chemicals, processed food and additives, and you don't know any better. Do yourself a favor, and have a go for a week. Or a day, and then make it two or more. Start with one day a week if you think a week is too much. Set one day a week, where you go clean, and keep it for a month, then add to it more days....

Many people eat very healthily and exercise their whole life and die of cancer at 50. Maybe sometimes it's just meant to be, or maybe sometimes people don't heal the soul but focus on the body. And any imbalance in our body or mind is going to have a negative effect on either the body or soul. Maybe it's destiny. None of us knows. But looking after your body will increase your chances and don't forget, you are going to feel good.

If you have an unhealthy relationship with food and it gives you negative emotions a few times a day, those emotions will be stored in your body, and it's not good for your overall health. Stress, guilt, anger, jealousy have a very negative impact on your body and mind. If your body is living in permanent stress, healthy eating will help a little, but more is needed. Change the way you think about yourself and your body and start having a more positive relationship with yourself.

When I trained clients, there was one thing that got me thinking a lot ...

I had to ask people at their initial assessment what medications they were taking, and I was shocked how many people were taking antidepressants, pills for anxiety, calming pills and stuff to help them sleep. Why do we overcook it so much? Is it social media, television, magazines, our unhealthy relationships or our unhealthy coping mechanisms? Answer this yourself ...

Many people in the media are psychopathic; they love to control minds. The media can be very nasty. How much do you let the media affect your mood? What happens when you see a food commercial on TV?

We were born without additives, without chemicals, without someone manipulating our way of thinking, and we were born healthy and perfect; why is it we go on to suffer mentally and physically?

How many people spend their lives doing what someone told them, or they live their lives as their families wish, as they are too scared to disappoint them? I am not surprised these days that people struggle and look for good feelings in food, as their life doesn't provide it anymore. Food and alcohol are great replacement.

FOR THE SOUL...

ALL THAT YOU HAVE IS YOUR SOUL

For many of us, how do or did we develop mental health problems?

1 in 6 people is dangerous for our mental health. I mentioned before, world is a shark's pool.

You are in a relationship with a sociopath. Who is going to develop mental health problems? Yes, you are. If I asked you to describe a sociopath, would you be able to? Some people spend their lives in a relationship with a sociopath, and they don't even know!

You are in a relationship with a narcissist. Who is going to develop mental health problems and sooner or later going to start having suicidal thoughts? Yes, you. Can you describe narcissist and narcissistic abuse? You surely will be able to describe it after you have experienced it, but would you know if you were going through the abuse, or would you accept you might be crazy?

You are bullied and being picked on at work or at home. Who is going to develop mental health problems? Yes, you. Do you bottle it up? What do you think happens with those suppressed emotions? I personally feel upset when people can see bullying taking place, and no one says a word. You are not crazy most people are too scared to say anything or do anything. Nobody wants to be a scapegoat.

You are going through emotional abuse. Are you already having anxiety issues? Are you going to struggle? Yes, you are.

How long have you been in this relationship? What stage is the frog at? Sometimes you cannot save the relationship or the other person unless they are willing to go to a qualified person and start sorting their problems out. But remember, the sociopath, narcissist and many other disordered characters won't go to a qualified person, as they are scared the therapist will see through them. But you can save yourself. Don't lose your strength. Sometimes you will be there emotionally for your partner, and sometimes your partner will be there for you, but if someone is using you constantly as an emotional punchbag you will suffer.

You have been abused for a long time, but you have learned to <u>make excuses</u> for people and have developed an addiction to it without even realizing it. Who is going to develop mental health problems? Do I need to ask?

10-15% of the population are on a moderate level of psychopathy. Oh, sorry, did you think psychopaths are in prison? No, but guess what, many victims are in prison as they snapped. Would you be able to describe how a psychopath functions? You did not realize that your charming amazing neighbour might be one of them?

Yes, we do miss lots of knowledge.

You used to be a happy individual, and you used to be confident. After a few years in this relationship your confidence has gone, you doubt yourself, you have outbursts of crying, you don't trust people, and you feel weirdly exhausted, and you are having dark thoughts? But you are doing everything right, and everything seems to be ok.

Maybe you were gaslighted to hell and back, and you don't even know this. Maybe the whole time you were dating an extremely charming sociopathic gas lighter, and you had no idea something was wrong ... dark thoughts are creeping up, and you are slowly starting to feel like maybe you are going crazy? You are in a relationship with a bad soul ... darling, save your soul ... there are so many great souls, but if you are a lovely soul, maybe you attract energy vampires as you are too nice? You could be the target. You are not a sandwich that people can have a bite from your soul. Eventually, nothing will be left, and you will become a walking shell.

You looked for love and self-validation in others, and you are getting exhausted as you cannot find it? Books on co-dependency, child neglect and its effect on a soul might start to make sense. Why we look for happiness in others, and why we get so hurt when people take us for granted. Maybe forget about people for a moment, and open the books with a glass of wine and put yourself first and read ... you might be surprised ... your soul needs healing.

If you are surrounded by people that lie to your face, people that don't respect boundaries, and people who manipulate you just to get something from you for their ego, who do you think is slowly going to experience anxiety and who is going to start having mental health problems ... ? Yes, you ...You can get addicted to your own toxic thoughts.... Be careful and pay attention to your thoughts. Make sure your wall is high to climb for toxic individuals. Remember, how do you feel after the person has left?

Do you know what causes depression in many cases? Lack of self-love. Some people give all their love and attention to others, and the person that they look at in the mirror gets nothing and keeps on giving. Needs are so overlooked that they end up depressed. Sometimes we are guilty of creating our own depression, but we need the ability to see it before it's too late. Otherwise, we can be in a dangerous situation for our mental health.

What I find the scariest is that a mental health problem creeps up without giving us a warning. That's the scary fact about it. And life can turn the heat up when you have a lot of stress, especially for a prolonged time. And then maybe one day you are sitting somewhere, and experience anxiety or a panic attack, and you have no idea what to do about it. And you wonder to yourself how it even happened. And then suddenly you have a problem, and you are not sure what to do with it or how to sort this problem out. It's scary. If you have good people around you, you have a good chance to sort it out, but if not, and you bottle it up, be careful. You can end up in a spiral.

If you're a loner that's not necessarily bad either, as you might reach for *books* and gain more *knowledge* than many friends would have.

If you compare yourself permanently with the lives of others or someone keeps comparing you … change your thinking, change your views, find a therapist to talk to and look after *your* well-being. You are good enough.

Let's learn to look after ourselves. Not just after the physical body, but also after the spiritual one. Both need our love and attention.

People who take our freedom away from us for their benefit are creators of mental health problems. Stress, abuse, our own coping mechanisms that we developed can be a cause of our problems. You can drive your own brain towards a fog where you slowly start losing the ability to think and see clearly.

Sometimes in life, you will hit rock bottom. Sometimes you have to break things completely to be able to fix them. Just never give up. Life is beautiful. Qualified people will help! But be picky, if one does not understand you, find a different one. It's your soul!

Many people will listen only to get control over you. Social services will fail you and many other authorities will fail you. Many people need a therapist, many find books and many just keep on going around and around until they can't anymore.

People can drive you crazy. Lack of knowledge can drive people crazy.

Sometimes we just need one thing: BREATHE FREELY AND BE TRUE TO OURSELVES.

I know it can be hard, and some people can be extremely difficult to deal with. But many books will give you guidance on how to deal with these individuals, and how to look after your own well - being.

Which pill are you taking in life? The red pill or the blue pill?

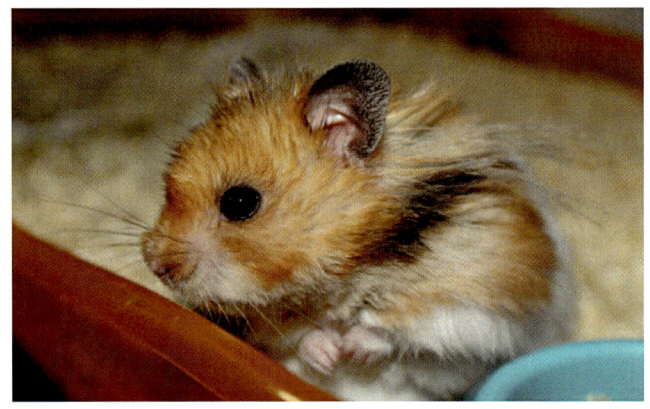

Chapter 7

HOW WE DO IT & BEAUTIFUL DREAMER

How do we do it then if we don't count calories?

Well, it's simple …

1) Eat healthily

2) Exercise daily

3) Practise mindfulness

4) Meditate daily for at least 20 minutes

5) Eat clean food

6) Take care of your mental and physical health

7) Have a hamster, so he reminds you to exercise daily

8) Surround yourself only with positive, nice people

9) Leave the job you hate

10) Get divorced

No worries, only kidding ☺

But if you follow at least 5? Congratulations

I will talk about exercise and how we do it, but if you don't exercise and many people don't, you can still be slim by following what I am going to explain when it comes to food. The reason, I would like you to exercise or go to yoga classes at least once a week is for your mental health. How exercise makes you feel due to the release of hormones and helps you to cope with stress is more important to me than what you look like.

Ok, if we do not count calories …

Some people just want to feel good or feel stronger. But let's be honest, most people want to reduce body fat. And the good news is, if you eat clean, your metabolism will speed up, so if you eat more clean than bad, you will lose body fat.

We look at client goals, and we take the measurements (we can measure body fat with callipers) and find out where our client is on the BMI scale (search BMI calculation).

Many people argue that "I have big muscles" or "heavy bones". Well, no, you don't have heavy bones, and yes, you have large muscles if you have to carry a body of 80kg compared to a 55kg body, so obviously, you're going to need bigger muscles to carry a bigger body around.

We ask what our client does for work, as it will give us an idea of how active or in-active the client is and what their fitness level will be. We really do not want to kill the client with the first session, with them crawling out of the gym or ending up sick in the bathroom, rather than happily walking out feeling enthused.

Remember, if you are just starting, don't make yourself feel sick by running like a hamster for a day or start lifting heavy weights right away, so you end up with a sore back and looking like an A&E candidate, as your fitness level is not ready to lift heavy. Find some workout that is going to make you feel good, and not like, "omg, this is going to kill me". Something will kill you one day, but it should not be exercise. About 15 people worldwide a year die of being stuck under the bench press as they get it too heavy, and they had no spotter to help them to finish their 'heavy' set. Don't be silly. If it is really hard, it's not right. If after your first session you are going to feel sick, what's the chance you're going to feel a little anxious coming back to the gym next time? This is your time, not "I am going to make myself sick" time.

We check for health conditions and if they are taking any medications. We do our research if we are not familiar with conditions and check for any previous injuries and limitations clients may have. Occasionally it's good to have a letter from their doctor to say people are medically fit to exercise. Remember, you are supposed to get stronger and leaner and not get yourself into a hospital. Know your body and know your condition. If you are not perfectly healthy, check.

We check what their daily diet is and their fluids intake, including alcohol. Once we know what we are working with, we know how the person is going to cope and start slowly making adjustments so the person will see results soon and feel better. We start to show how to take the exit from the roundabout the client has been on for years when it comes to food and dieting. Normally, changes are slow, but some people really want to go hard for it, so you change their diet and hope their addictions are not going to be stronger than their desire.

It is all about cutting down on processed foods and foods that are more difficult for your body to break down.

We check if there are types of exercise the client likes or dislikes, as you don't want to kill someone mentally and physically on a treadmill if they clearly tell you they hate running.

If you are having a stressful day at work and home, for example, and then you are supposed to go to the gym, which you hate, what's the point? You will be mentally breaking yourself. Having a stressful day and looking forward to the workout or jumping on a bike for an hour after work as you need to switch off is a great thing you can do to de-stress. If it's yoga or pilates or any other slow workout, but you feel good after it, the job is done. It's supposed to be a joy or a catch up with a friend.

After we have checked for goals, we give clients realistic feedback, as to tell someone they can lose in a healthy way 20 kgs of body fat in a month is clearly unrealistic and a lie.

Most people have been through an emotional roller coaster with diets, so once they hear it's doable to have long term success, and get to the point where they need to be, it's more satisfying for them than telling them some crazy diet works. Sometimes people are a bit disappointed, as they are expecting some magic pill and it means they will have to put real effort in. There is no magic weight loss pill …

Many people believe "if I was slim, I would be happy". If I was 60kgs, I would be happy. Remember, if your main goal is a number, it's not going to be as nice as if you genuinely learn to like your body and soul. It will be a more pleasurable journey. And the habit will stay for life potentially. If you do it for a number, you will easily return back to your old habits, and the weight will come back whilst you're not looking.

Food diary

- It helps people realize their eating patterns, habits, builds self-awareness of intake (many people while on the phone to their friends manage to eat a whole bag of sweets, and then later on completely forget about it!).

- It helps us to see what needs to be changed or adjusted, and it shows us where the problems are. Once we have the knowledge, it's very simple to see.

- We introduce a client to smiley faces to record how they feel 30 minutes after eating food. Why 30 minutes? As I introduced you to insulin response and metabolism earlier, the body will tell you how it feels. Either it goes on strike, would love to tell you off and have an argument, wants to get divorced or feels happy with you. How you feel is the answer, but you mostly don't pay attention to it as your attention is focused on the immediate happy feeling while you were eating, and you don't pay attention to how you feel after 30 minutes. The food diary will remind you to have a think. You will be surprised.

- How much sugar and carb intake you have.
- Overeating or undereating of calories.

Some people have a mentally wrong approach, as they hear the word diet, and they automatically hear the word suffer.

Remember, many people hear the word change, and they also feel uneasy. Diet is simply your daily intake of food. And change is good! You are here to change things as the old things did not or do not serve you anymore, and the old things are making you ill. Change is good and no one is asking you to suffer or be unhappy. You might be so used to the roundabouts and ups and downs that you can't imagine your life without them.

Why do you think so many people become addicted to fitness, exercise and a healthier lifestyle? They realize how good it makes them feel, so the good feeling is their new high.

Isn't it great to feel good mentally and physically? You might have to check your beliefs and habits, as they might also be your limitations. Do you say to yourself, I am never going to be slim or, I am a failure? Or do you feel mentally strong, you can achieve anything?

One more thing I want to stress. I cannot see any reason why people should be eating food they don't like or food that does not taste good to them. It's nonsense. There is so much to choose from.

The only problem you might have is to do a little bit of research or occasionally cook. That's all. There is so much to choose from, and social media is full of recipes. Be creative.

The positive side is that once you adjust your food, your taste buds are going to be livelier as they are also getting out of the drugged state from sugar, heavily processed foods and additives, so food is going to start being delicious, as it's meant to taste.

How do we adjust food diary and food intake?

- You can see from all the above that to change diet too quickly is not advisable as most of us are so highly addicted to food and many people, especially when stressed, return to their old habits.

- What is the most important meal for a person? For some lunch, some dinner. You leave this meal to last for making changes, in case it's an unhealthy choice. If someone says lunch is most important, then you change breakfast for one week. Or you can alternate. One day the person changes breakfast, next day, they revert back to their habitual breakfast. Mind you, it takes a little time for a person to get out of habits and make a change. You want to do it slowly, so it's not too stressful for people, but more fun and a nice change. People need time to adjust and change. You know yourself how hard it is to change your habit.

- Remember, food is a joy! Not punishment or something that is supposed to give you negative emotions. Make sure you like the taste of your new food!

- Each week, you make more changes. You look at how the client is (be your own client) dealing with it. How do you feel mentally? Missing something, or I feel better? Focus on a positive! Feeling better, and my new breakfast tastes really nice, AND I don't need to worry about calories or gaining fat, as with clean food, my body will struggle to store it as fat; it's going to use it as healthy fuel and nutrition. I don't need to feel guilty for eating; I can enjoy my food.

- Small steps, so you hardly notice, but you feel better.

- So, let's say, we have changed breakfast for the first week, and it's ok. Next week in addition we alternate, and one day we change lunch, and the next day dinner.

- If you prefer you can choose to change 5 meals a week the first week, then 8, then 10 and what suits you. If you are having snacks for the first week, you can only change snacks, and next week change snacks plus breakfast. You should feel good with your pace. Have a think where you want to start. You are making choices and changes for yourself.

- You are slowly getting rid of bad food, and addictions are not driving you over the edge. Taste is slowly coming back, and you should by now feel much better. A few pounds might be off as well. If you exercise on top of this, you're going to have some weight loss, but it depends, as of course many people start to exercise, and they put 2kgs on. Don't forget muscle is heavier than fat, so you will initially be losing inches rather than weight. Have a look at the difference between a lean 58 kg female versus a 58 kg average female without as much lean muscle. And remember, your body might hold onto fat for a few weeks, as you intoxicated it so badly with diet roundabouts it's a bit drunk and needs a little time to sober up.

- After around 3 weeks, a client (or you) should feel much better as you slowly exchange your meals. Remember, NO ONE eats good always. If you remember my talk earlier about metabolism, if you eat some bad food it can deal with it so long as you don't overload it. Do not drive yourself crazy – I MUST not eat this. It's going to have the opposite effect and create guilt and a roller coaster of cravings.

- People will start to enjoy their new eating regime, and then you can easily apply the 80% good, 20% bad, formula and still have weight loss. You don't have to go exactly 80% and 20% but start eating cleaner with less processed food, and you are winning. It depends on how much a person wants to be good and how quickly they want to see results.

- But remember that weight loss stops every few weeks, sometimes for two weeks, as your body thinks you are trying to kill it. It desperately holds the weight for a while as it's scared for your well-being. Ignore it.

- *If you do a calorie deficit,* remember when you have lost around 5kg, do the calculation again and create another small deficit. A smaller body needs a smaller number of calories, and a bigger body needs a larger number. Imagine your body as a car fuel tank. A big heavy car is going to use more fuel than a small one. It's logic.

- We are slowly getting a person to change habits towards clean eating. Because clean eating has great benefits for metabolism, insulin response and weight loss. It is easier than counting calories as well. Celebrities with a magic weight loss are clean eating and exercising once or twice a day; it just depends on how much "magic" they are after.

- Remember 70% is food and 30% exercise. We don't like to tell this to clients as they will stop exercising as much as they otherwise would have, and some will cancel their gym membership. There is this myth where people say she got her body through such hard work. Well, hang on a minute, if you don't enjoy spending time exercising and you are not feeling better after exercising, you won't last. It's not hard work, it's a healthy choice.

- Sugar plus carbs together are a killer for your diet. If you eat them more often than you should, your weight is going to creep up.

- The cleaner you eat the more weight you lose. My clients generally lose more than the recommended guidelines when they start. The great thing is they feel better, their skin and sleep improve, and they are more positive.

- You become healthier and more balanced when it comes to your body.
- Food starts to taste like food and not as chemicals or sugars. The cleaner you are eating, the more you will be noticing that lots of food doesn't taste as good as you used to think, but you will become more ''addicted'' to healthier food. Processed food is going to start to feel heavy, and you will have noticed from your food diary how much food has an effect on you.
- You will be losing weight without a massive effort and still eating enjoyably.
- You will become more aware of your feelings, and it might help in your personal life as well, as sometimes we become numb to toxicity as we have got used to it.
- Self-care will be a pleasure as you will notice that it's not so difficult to have the body you want.
- Remember the power of 3. If you make changes, the first 3 days are the hardest. After 3 days it becomes much easier, and a new routine is being created. Or your first 3 food changes might be the hardest. Then it becomes easier.

DAILY FOOD DIARY

	MO	TU	WED	TH	FR	SAT	SUN
BREAKFAST							
LUNCH							
DINNER							
SNACKS							
SMILEY FACES							
ACTIVITY							
FEELINGS							

Under activity, write what kind of exercise you do.

Feelings: After a meal. Did you feel like you are missing something? What are your addictions? Mentally pay attention. Practise self-awareness.

Smiley faces: set a timer for **30 minutes** after your meal and write down how you feel. Tired, happy, heavy. That's when your body will tell you how food makes you feel in the longer term.

FOR THE SOUL...

BEAUTIFUL DREAMER

Was one of your parents an alcoholic?

The inner child of a child who had an alcoholic parent ...

Do you remember your childhood and your inner talk? Some do not, and some people's childhood affected them more than it should. Maybe some in negative ways and maybe some in positive ones.

Many children feel through their childhood feelings of confusion, vulnerability, shame, guilt, fear, anxiety and insecurity, and many develop symptoms of PTSD as adults.

If one of your parents was alcoholic, maybe you are having some of these things going on …

Some common feelings children of alcoholics might experience

Children of alcoholics can have problems in intimate relationships, feelings of being different from other people, can overreact to changes over which they have no control, are either super responsible or super irresponsible, some can have a problem to say the truth and rather lie, can take themselves too seriously, constantly seek approval and affirmation, have difficulties to guess what is normal and what isn't.

Many children of alcoholics didn't have much fun or had no fun at all. The inner child is wounded, and if a person does not seek help, they can struggle their whole life. Many took the role of an adult, and became super responsible. Those little adult children. Maybe they smiled a lot, but no one knew how hurt they were inside. They could feel things rather more than most people around, but there was no one who could see it.

For some kids being at home was like being in hell. They could not wait to grow up and be gone. But for now, they were trapped, and they had to teach themselves coping mechanisms that no one told them about. These coping mechanisms can become a danger in adult life. Some coping strategies that kids develop are not healthy in the long term.

Some become super-achievers or overachievers in adult life. And many end up with break downs or burnouts as they did not learn to look after themselves, and they simply put everything and everyone ahead of themselves. Can you see how dangerous it is if we didn't heal our childhood wounds?

Some did not do well at school. They struggled with concentration. They were preoccupied with fantasies about their life being ok and daydreaming. No one really cared how they did at school. Many times they cried for help, but no one was there.

Friendships might have been hard, as they always felt a little different and kind of an outsider. They struggled to believe someone actually liked them. Having fun was pretty difficult for them as the child in them was so repressed.

If your parent was an alcoholic: Do you remember? What was your inner talk?

"One day, I am going to buy myself a house, which is going to be mine, and I will be safe there."

"One day, I will have a family that loves me and will never abandon me?"

"I am going to make sure I never end up in a relationship with an alcoholic?"

"One day, I am going to have people around me that love me and are kind and fun?"

"I am not loveable and good enough, but one day I will find someone who is going to love me?"

"As soon as I can, I will leave this home, as I feel like I am in their way all the time and they are unhappy because I was born?"

"I was somehow accidentally born here, and one day I'm going to find out if I was adopted or not and maybe find the family that loves me?"

"Once I grow up, I will spend the rest of my life making up for what I did not have, to make up for it."

Many of these are the normal thinking processes of children of alcoholics.

Possibly they never learnt the healthy self - love they need and are looking for happiness, sometimes in the wrong relationships. Many of them marry alcoholics or end up becoming one. Something known to them: a false sense of security. They don't like change, and 'normal' relationships can be terrifying for them as it's unfamiliar. They can be terrified of personal criticism and fear people, and authority figures as they never received positive validation, and criticism can make them more vulnerable towards a feeling of low self-esteem. They struggle with intimate relationships, as they are too scared of abandonment. Many end up depressed.

The adult was constantly leaving them, as alcohol was number one, so fear of abandonment subconsciously looms large. Many children of alcoholics, therefore, have a problem leaving abusive relationships.

There is one big positive that you maybe don't realize. You have already been through hell, so don't live in it anymore. Possibly you have suppressed emotional traumas that can be relieved through therapy. You can function alone, and you will be a more independent person than most people around you.

Functioning alone won't be a problem for you, and when problems come, you will be more capable of finding solutions than most people around you, but you will be fighting the feeling you are not good enough and possibly self - doubt will be knocking at the door.

When you are in a relationship, you have been so used to a chaotic family and constant drama that you might find it difficult to relax in the relationship and not to be always waiting for a battle. You are possibly addicted to that stress without realising it.

Remember, no organism can live in constant stress; it's very unhealthy for your body and mind. It is asking for illnesses. To be healthy and happy, we need to heal.

We were not born to suffer and struggle.

Emotionally and mentally, we possibly got addicted to stress from living in those environments, but we did not know it. You might not even know that you are constantly stressed as it became your natural state. Prolonged stress becomes an addiction.

If you have gone through therapy and now live the life you always wanted, you will have more gratitude for a calm life and when things go well. Many people don't appreciate these things.

You are fully aware that now that it's your life, you can make yourself happy with your choices, but you might be a little scared and almost feel guilty for being happy or successful.

To heal your inner child is important for the happiness you want.

You've already had it tough, now it's time to do it your way and be happy. The therapy many therapists use is CBT (Cognitive Behavioural Therapy), as we might have developed unhealthy coping mechanisms that can do more harm later on.

I have no experience with CBT therapy, but it's well known by therapists and it help you understand how your thoughts, beliefs, and attitudes affect your behaviour and feelings and teach you healthy coping skills.

EMDR therapy, meditation, self-care and knowing why you feel the way you do and learning new paths of self-valuation and love are very important for your healing. It can be very emotional, painful, but also a beautiful journey. Your gratitude will give you some amazing feelings once you are healed.

If you were to read a book on children of alcoholics, is there anything you can lose except gaining knowledge? Can it help you and open your eyes?

Maybe lead to a healthier life? What do you want? Fix it or live in survival mode?

Some say it's our DNA. No, it's important when it comes to medical care as it will be a factor, but the choices we make in life shape us to who we are later on. It's a choice. To heal or suffer. To seek help or live as a victim in self-pity. The choice is yours.

At the end, I will put a list of books that I hope might help. Many might be hard to read, but when you become more aware of your unhealthy coping patterns, there's more chance you can slowly change them. If it's abuse, many of these books explain how to answer the abuser and how to protect yourself. It will be hard to be in control, and not fall back to your old ways, but when you manage to stay in control, you will be gaining self-respect, control over your life and slowly stop accepting abuse.

Sometimes, we are traumatized, and we lie to ourselves and to others around as we are scared of the truth. When you are ready, face the truth and heal. There is no joy, without pain.

Chapter 8)

FAST CAR & MY RED PILL THERAPY

This sports car of yours.

What does your sports car need? Fuel and oil. Your body is your vehicle which takes you from A to B, and it needs the same. But if you put bad fuel into your sports car, what is going to happen? It's not good, is it? The same for your body.

Let's keep it simple.

Let's say you wake up in the morning, and you stand up. Your muscles are getting to work. What do you need for your muscles? PROTEIN. (Fuel)

Your bones and joints to keep healthy and your metabolism to work? FAT (Oil)

What about carbohydrates? A typical argument is that you need carbohydrates …. well, you can get your carbs from vegetables, don't forget. You will also get lots of other vitamins and minerals from vegetables, fruits and whole foods.

I am going to introduce you to clean eating. At first, it might be a little confusing, but once you understand it, there are lots of foods to choose from.

It's hard these days, as additives are added a lot. Remember 80% good and 20% bad. This is how fitness people do it. You can eat much worse than 80% good and still be ok, as it depends on how active you are or how good you are with food and self-awareness.

If you are not a gym goer 6 days a week, you don't need to worry. It still works, but it's up to you how fast you will get results, as it simply depends on how long it's going to take you to make adjustments or how passionate you will become about looking after yourself a little bit more.

In a later chapter, there will be my week of clean eating for you, but I am going to be honest, I only managed this once for a week, and since then, I have been trying but never made it again fully, as I have two or three coffees a day, too much cheese, and many toffee cream meringues, but I am still 70% good most days.

I strongly recommend you try clean eating for a week, as after a week I felt amazing. Up until then, I hadn't realized it was possible to feel so good. At least once in your lifetime, go for it and see the difference.

What do I mean by clean eating?

Everything that is (ideally) organic, without additives, not processed and not cooked at high temperatures. No food that is genetically modified or food where animals were treated with antibiotics or hormones. Eat for a week with the minimum toxicity possible, with the minimum of chemicals and additives, and most food should be organic.

You are going to have to do a bit of cooking. No alcohol at all if possible, and drink 8 glasses of either water or fruit tea without sugar daily. For sweetener, only use organic honey, no sugar, no brown sugar and no artificial sweeteners.

Don't worry, I will give you some examples later. It massively stabilises your whole body, and your metabolism is going to love you for this. You will sleep well, feel rested, your skin is going to improve, and your whole body will start to recover from years of toxins and additives.

It's up to you if you want to do it right away or take a few days and make some changes before you feel ready to go for it 100%.

You will not be able to go completely clean, as it's nearly impossible these days, as the wind blows some small amounts of chemicals that have been sprayed onto organic crops.

So, what do we mean by changing nutrition to go cleaner? Eat more stuff that is easier for your digestive system to process. Imagine it as everything nature gives you without humans putting too much effort into it. It's easier than you might think.

I had a couple of clients and friends that asked me how and what to eat. Most of them came back and told me they lost 5kg in the first month without any additional exercise. And yes, it's doable ok. The moment they start clean eating along with exercising, results are fast.

I had a housemate who lost 12 kgs in a year with no exercise. She just changed her diet a little and enjoyed clean eating. But she was a bit of a party animal, so clean eating often went hand in hand with alcohol, and as you can imagine, most of us humans, after we drink alcohol, we will eat whatever is in our way and more. But if you change things and maintain a bit of a balance between good and bad, you will be ok. If you can do better than bad, you will be winning. It's as simple as that. Just as in life, the goal is the balance, as we all have to deal with bad periods sometimes. Life is not always good ...

Another client of mine wanted to go for it right away, without slow changes, and there are many people who are happy to do this, as they are mentally strong when it comes to food. After nearly two months of mostly clean eating, on her night out, she had her favourite takeaway and promptly threw up, as she found it disgusting. Your taste cells will change if you start clean eating, and your body will let you know what it doesn't want anymore. You will not feel good after heavily processed food. You will enjoy the taste of real food so much more, it will be like an awakening for you. Remember the power of 3. Either the first 3 meals, 3 days or 3 weeks will be difficult. Then it will get easier. It will be more of a new habit.

I am sure you have wondered how some celebrities do it when they hire a personal trainer, and then they have a massive weight loss in a year. It's very simple. Firstly, they must decide in their head they're going to do it, as this is half the battle. Then they start clean eating, and with workouts 1-2 times a day, they create a calorie deficit. Their cravings will be high, but it's much easier to keep it under control with the right knowledge. They eat frequently, so the body keeps working and cravings are more under control, and their metabolism is high. I am sure you will have noticed many do lots of running. Why? Because it's the quickest way to lose weight. Your whole body is working, and by running for 20 minutes and more, you will speed up your metabolism for another 24 hours. It's as simple as that.

It's a lot about self-control, self-awareness, self-discipline and the right knowledge.

If your new clean diet is as colourful and as tasty as possible, the cravings for sugar and processed carbs won't be as crazy.

Benefits of clean eating

- If you eat clean, you will probably be eating at home, as you have to prepare the food, which will be more enjoyable than eating a burger in a car.
- Your taste cells will lose their addiction to the flavour enhancers, and you will taste so much more. You can practise eating like Hemingway
- You will live longer and your health is going to improve significantly
- Your body will function smoothly, and your brain will function better
- You will have more energy and you are going to sleep much better than you have been used to
- Sex is going to be much better according to studies (have fun)
- Benefits for the planet
- Your body will become stronger
- Your mood is going to improve

- You will start losing weight without too much effort
- Lower inflammation
- Skin, hair and nails are going to improve
- Faster recovery after your workouts
- <u>Stronger immune system</u>
- <u>Better mental health</u>
- Less cravings for unhealthy food
- Less sugar addiction
- Less chronic pain
- Save money
- Sustainable healthy lifestyle
- Better focus
- … and many more

Try it strictly for one week, and you will experience how good you feel, and then you will be more motivated to stay with clean eating.

You might get a little emotional if you start researching additives, chemicals and sugar. You will wonder if the food manufacturers are trying to slowly kill us, but the anger will help you to make changes.

What should you cook with?

I recommend for cooking use: Organic whenever you can.

- Organic butter
- Cold - pressed oils
- Coconut oil
- Olive oil
- Lard (but less)

When it comes to milk and dairy

- For your week of clean eating, you should use organic full fat or half fat milk. Many people use coconut milk, cashew milk, almond milk, but many of these are in cartons with added chemicals for long life. For your week of clean eating, you should use products without any additives.
- Milk products. If you like yoghurts, it should be full fat Greek organic yoghurt and any type of fruit with a spoonful of organic honey if you have a sweet tooth.
- Cheese. If you can, go organic (it's harder to find sometimes) and remember, that your daily portion of cheeses should be the size of a matchbox for this week. Milk should be a small cup a day (in case you make a smoothie, you might overshoot it, so have different types of healthy breakfast if possible).
- Avoid all low-fat products or any reduced calorie products as many of them have lots of sweeteners and additives to ensure

taste, as everything was sucked out of them to reduce calories, but they are also very low in nutrients, and your metabolism simply needs fat.

Meat or if you are a vegetarian or vegan

- All meat and eggs should be organic. Your weekly intake should be two oily fish a week. Make sure they are fresh and organic. Look at the back of shelves in the shops, as meat or salmon that are fresh are put at the back, as supermarkets need to sell the older products first; check the dates!

Fluids and drinks

- For your week of clean eating, fluids should be water, tea, if possible organic. Many tea bags have been bleached. If they have a white colour, you will notice the difference if you buy organic teabags. Another option is to tear the bag or buy loose tea.
- Water, still or sparkling
- Homemade iced tea
- One cup of coffee a day
- Homemade fruit juice

Fruits and vegetables

- All fresh and organic.

- If you can't always get organic, don't worry too much, but remember always wash your fruit and veg.
- No one was ever diagnosed with illness from eating too much fruit and veg. Try different fruits and vegetables; have a play. Try different recipes as you might discover a new favourite food. There are hundreds of recipes with fruits and veg that you will never have tried before. People have a tendency to overthink it and overcomplicate it as they try to follow the clean eating guidelines. There is no guarantee you're not going to be diagnosed with a disease. But we can minimize our chances, and we only have this body, and we should look after it. It's your only car for this lifetime.

Breakfast clean eating

One coffee a day is ok. One a day will give you a boost and wake you up.

Coffee should be of good quality, organic if possible. If you have milk, it should be organic milk and full fat. If that's too much, semi-skimmed milk with reduced fat is ok, but if you can avoid skimmed milk as it has got no nutrients (you would be better off having a glass of water).

If you have a fruit juice it must be freshly squeezed, don't use bottles or cartons, as they have additives to keep them drinkable for longer, plus possibly added sugar or sweeteners.

If you drink tea and normally use sugar or sweeteners, you must replace it with honey, (maple syrup) or have nothing. If you drink black tea with milk, the milk should be full fat or reduced fat milk and organic honey (remember your daily allowance is a small mug of milk).

You should drink 6-8 glasses of water a day. Your fluid intake should be around 2 litres a day. If you don't like water, try a pint of water with fruits in, as it will give the water a sweet taste. Blueberries, strawberries, oranges, apples, whatever you like and then after you have drunk the water you can eat the fruit. Double benefit; water and fruit!

Other options are fruit teas, as some people struggle to drink water. There are many options in the shops; look at what flavour you might like and enjoy. There are a number of teas to choose from around the world, and it's fun to try different flavours. There are many herbal teas as well, but you need to look further than a standard supermarket. Have a nice walk around town and find new places.

Find the taste YOU LOVE! That will mean you will get your income of liquids! Have fun with it and enjoy it. Try new tastes, new things; don't get stuck with the old stuff. New is more exiting! Have fun! Black tea can dehydrate, so it's not recommended you have more than one or two cups a day.

For one week, no alcohol, no pre-packed fruit juices, coke, or any sweetened drinks.

No processed carbs for one week.

All carbs should be sweet potatoes, vegetables, whole foods.

Remember, many vegetables have carbs in as well, so you are not missing out on them. Some people feel that if they don't eat carbs, something is wrong, as carbs give them the feeling of being full …

Many people go into panic mode thinking that if they don't get stuffed with processed carbs, they are going to die, as they are used to having that satisfied feeling that carbs give you. If you are one of them, have a good portion of lentils or veg or sweet potato.

Salt and pepper can be used and herbs and spices, but no stocks or flavour enhancers. If you can, use Himalayan salt.

Snacks should not be "healthy" bars (to hold the bar together, they must have added something to stick it together). Remember, 20% of food labelling is not accurate, and many things don't have to be put on the labels, so we go clean this week, as clean as possible. Whole foods, either dried fruits, peanuts, seeds; explore. Many dried fruits mixes are great and very tasty. A great snack is a spoonful of peanut butter. Great for a straight source of protein. Also helps with cravings. Don't eat the whole jar; eat a spoonful (it's a snack, not lunch, have a tablespoonful, if you had a meltdown and ate the whole jar don't have anything else). Avocados, bananas, blueberries (great for your brain if you work in an office). Whole foods. Carrots with hummus. Go and have a look and find something you like and have not had for ages. Or have something new!

If you have an allergy to peanuts, snack on fruits. A snack is half an avocado, 2 slices of parma ham or dried fruit. All sizes should be a handful for snacks and for normal meals the size of an average plate. Don't over complicate it. If you fail with one meal, it's not such a tragedy but TRY clean eating for a week once in your life to see the effect on you and how you feel. A difference in your way of thinking about food and self-care will mentally help you.

Many of my clients make a very basic mistake. They change their breakfast and start to have porridge. Let me explain to you, as I have had this conversation rather too often with people. Porridge is healthy but not good if you are losing weight. Why? Simply because when you have porridge, you will realize that it takes you much longer before you get hungry. You also feel fuller when you have had porridge. It means one thing; your porridge is too heavy for your digestive system, and porridge is a slow release of energy, which means before your body has a chance to break it and use it, it's already tired as it was hard work. It slows down the metabolism.

Lunch and dinners

Lots of vegetables. If you like chicken or meat, they should be organic. Salads, any kind you like.

If you use dressings, have a look at homemade ones and have fun making them. There are lots of options. You are doing this for your body and soul. Have a new experience.

Try to make it as colourful as you possibly can. If there is something, you really like such as broccoli or asparagus or any kind of fruit or veg, great. Your body is probably telling you that you are missing some nutrient that is present in this food. Don't be scared to go with it. I have met people who literally lived on kale, broccoli, and rocket salads nearly their whole lives and they are in good health. But make it as colourful and interesting, but balanced, as you can. Learn to eat food, real food.

The great thing is if you do clean eating for two meals a day and you have one meal which is not great, your body can still manage to work with it, so there is no point in feeling guilty. But that's after you have done your week of clean eating.

Just enjoy it. Enjoy the change and pay attention to how you feel mentally and how your body responds to food and changes.

The mental effect will be more visible to you. In my example week, I will help explain what to use for cooking and what clean eating is about.

FOR THE SOUL...

MY RED PILL THERAPY

You might have noticed that I have mentioned EMDR therapy a few times in the book.

With the agreement of a dear friend, who has been through some difficult times, I am going to share her experience with EMDR therapy.

This is her story ...

When I was 35, I had a number of stressful life events, one after another, that were just too much. They left me in a state where I lost all my strength and the will to keep going. I was exhausted mentally and physically.

I overcooked myself so much that most people and friends around me thought I was on my way out.

I hardly slept for nearly two years. I developed a number of physical problems. I felt numb, and I was just a living shell and lost all the feelings I used to have. I felt nothing.

I was too nice. I had no boundaries, I made too many excuses for nasty people, and never put myself first in my life. Took lots of abuse at work, suffered a physical attack, and had to deal with some nasty people as well as abusive members of my family for years, and then at the end, to top it all off, with a cheating fiancée and the death of a close friend. It was all too much, and it was all happening at the same time.

But I thought I was ok. I didn't see my breakdown coming, as I always managed to forgive, move on and be that better person. Now I think I was a stupid person that was missing lots of knowledge on abuse and self-care.

I had got myself into a relationship, and I was supposed to get married. I was happy. I lived the dream for a while. For the first time in my life, I was excited and planned to spend the rest of my life with someone I loved deeply and adored. I thought finally, I am going to have a family I never had.

I was wrong.

Things went so wrong, and after a very nasty break up, I was done. Everything I had ever bottled up suddenly jumped out at me, and I realized that to clean this mess up was mission impossible. I was always strong, at least that's how I'd felt, but somehow, suddenly, I was down on my knees, and to getting up every morning became my hardest battle. I was the frog, and the water was coming to the boil …

I developed a persistent cough that was so nasty that waitresses would bring me a glass of water when I was in pubs and asked if I was ok. People would look at me with pity, and they seemed to be looking at someone who would soon be gone. I did not see how bad it was. I saw it in people's faces, but not in the mirror. I still kept telling myself, you will get through, you'd got through worse in life.

I had had hard times, but I never paid too much attention to it, as I believed I was a strong individual, and believed that I was a good person, and I am going to be ok. I always tried to do the right thing, but I did not realize that maybe my strength was my biggest weakness. And doing the right thing was the right thing for others, but not for me.

Things went so wrong that I thought to myself, no one could survive this. My strength was gone.

I was choking throughout the night and day, I was shaking 24 hours a day, I was having funny visions, but I blamed it on lack of sleep. I started to have a bluish colour that people have when they die, I struggled to function, getting up was too much, eating was making me feel sick, and sleeping was more some kind of shaking in bed, looking at the empty dark space.

Do you know what the best thing was when you are tied to a bed, and you can't get up? The only thing you can do there is breathe. I thought that's it. I am done. My body was too tired to sleep, and too tired to get up. I was lying there for a couple of hours, and I looked back at my life. Happy times, a stronger than life person that was fighting her battles and everyone else's battles. Fearless and full of dreams. Always full of ambitions and an animal lover that travelled the world. I thought of my dreams, and I thought this is not what was supposed to happen? I am not done yet! I wanted to do so much more, and I still had my dreams.

What helped? Do you know when they always say we have a dark side, and people talk about demons? I never knew about them, but now I started to feel them. They started to get angry, and I believe they saved my life. I had a few uncontrolled outbursts, and I screamed my face off at people that were nasty to me. I finally stood up for myself, and my last bits of strength were my outbursts at the nasty people who had got me into this position. I had never felt better in my life getting it out of my body. I knew I was dealing with some nasty stuff, but I used to shrug my shoulders and be that better person. Screaming at a few individuals felt amazing, and frankly they deserved it.

It felt like I was gone, but my body was still functioning. Every morning was such a battle that suddenly to get up became the hardest task in my life.

Most days, I could not get up, as I lost all my strength and my body became so weak I had to roll over on the side of the bed and put my knees on the floor and get up. Even this started to be too difficult.

I burst into tears to my friend and said, I just can't go on anymore, I am finished, but my body is still going. I was so exhausted I was nearly begging my body to let me go, as I couldn't pull through this.

In bed, I had time to think. How have I managed to get to this point in life, and into this bed?

How did I get here?

Things started to be clear, and I saw every person that had given me a kick over the years and slowly put me into this place. Maybe it was me, as I realized my coping mechanisms and poor boundaries got me here, as I was always trying to see the good in people, and lied to myself as I did not want to see the truth.

People talk about demons, but I've seen more demons in people that got me on my knees than demons inside of me. And the demons inside were slowly getting angry as more and more I was realizing the truth of how I got there.

I started to be angry with myself and with people that were just nasty. People that I would call demons. I was aware of my awakening feelings but also scared. I knew I had not done everything for the best, but I knew I was more capable and genuine than many of the people I had met.

I knew I was not a bad person.

Maybe releasing these demons and having a go at the people that were nasty to me saved my life. My demons kicked in, and they were on the rampage. They did not let me fall.

There is a song from Hozier, Arsonist's Lullaby, where he says, "never tame your demons, but keep them on a leash". Somehow the demons inside me were my lifesavers. You need to get it out, otherwise, the explosion inside will kill you and the nasty people's demons will win. Screaming helps, sometimes.

One evening I exploded and cried to my friend that I just could not take anymore. He suggested I talk to his girlfriend and ask her, as she goes to some lady and she helps her a lot. In a few days, I met up with his girlfriend and asked her who she goes to.

That was the start of my recovery. This lady did reiki. I had nothing to lose. I was so exhausted, I would do anything. I would frankly have preferred to die as my exhaustion was too much, and

I could not see the way out of this. And I had lost pretty much everything as well.

I went to this lady, and when I was lying on the table, my body went into a strange cramp. I was not able to move my hands as I felt something going through my body. I nearly threw up. I had a massive pain around my head and stomach, and my hands were paralysed.

I struggled to eat as I felt constantly sick, but after this session, I was so hungry I ate like a horse. I was so hungry and thirsty, like never before in my life. I went to a shop, bought two pizzas, cooked them both, ate them and drank so much tea and water that night that it was unreal.

This was the first time in two years when I slept soundly. After this sessions, I realized my body was starting to recover, but I also realized I had so much to fix that all I wanted to do was cry. And I did a lot. It helped. Every day for months.

After a few more outbursts, I called my friend, a psychologist, and told her I lost my temper a few times and screamed my face off at some people.

She said with massive relief in her voice, thank God for this, and congratulations. I said, you must explain this as I think I am going mad.

She said after I spoke to her some time back, she knew I had two choices. I will either break and scream and go a little wild and stand up for myself and choose the path of a healthy person that decides to save herself or bottle it up, and the explosion inside will kill me or get me really badly sick, and I will end up dead sooner than I would wish for.

I was shocked after hearing this. I also knew what she meant. I knew we could talk, but the hard work was going to be over to me, and I was scared.

But after screaming at a few people, I felt like, Jesus this feels so good, I could get

used to it … don't worry, I am back to normal these days.

I realized that many things in my life were not right, and I had no other option than to start fixing things. But how? It was such a mess. I called my friend and asked her to recommend some books, as I struggled to trust people. It was people that got me into this bed. I felt unsafe in the presence of people. It was hard. I was reading and reading, and I could see my errors, and everything started to make sense.

I started therapy as I wanted to know how to fix it all, but I soon realized that therapy did not help, and I had already spoken about stuff so many times to some of my friends that I did not want to talk about it anymore.

But my biggest problem was that I felt like something in my brain had changed, and I was not able to fix it, and I was aware that therapy was not going to help.

I totally overcooked it and did not see how to fix it. I was scared.

I went too far, I did not trust anyone at all, I doubted my own reality and being surrounded by people was scary, and I could not relax.

I worked on recovery so much and so hard, but the improvements I saw were too slow. I read countless psychology books and came to understand how I got to where I had got to.

I was doing better, but I knew I still had a problem. I started to get really worried about how to fix this. People around me were telling me I was looking so much better, but I knew something was not right, and I was scared. Really scared.

I was having dark thoughts of what if I can't fix myself?

I was sharing a house with a friend who told me about his boss who had had such a terrible time that he ended up in hospital for two weeks when he exhausted himself so much his body failed him, and he became unconscious. I thought seriously someone managed to take it further than me? My friend told me his boss had helped a colleague (a girl), and her story was very similar to mine. After working with him, it was unreal to see how she improved. I was desperate to meet him as I hoped he could point me in the right direction.

I did, but we never spoke about the problem, and we talked about other stuff. But I had a really good feeling about what he did. I knew he had a stressful job, and he was occasionally seeing a psychologist. I realized that many people in high positions have a psychologist on the side, as the stress can be overwhelming, and unless people can learn to de-stress and have good coping mechanisms it's hard to cope.

I messaged him and asked him if he knew a good psychologist who could help?

His therapist was too busy, but she managed to recommend me to her friend and thank God for that, as she, fortunately, did not do "talk therapy". This lady was nicely full - on (she gave me impression of I knowing what she was doing), and we spoke for a while, and then she just told me to "follow my fingers". She introduced me to a therapy called EMDR, and after my first session, I am not going to lie, I thought I was going to die again. My next day, and my third day were so brutal that I hated her, and the guy who recommended me to her as it was just too much.

I had no idea what was going on, but it was unreal.

I told myself never ever again, I just can't cope. But on the fifth day, I woke up, and I felt like I had not felt for many years. I straight away messaged her and asked her can you book me in again ASAP?

She did, and when I got to her, she said, how do you feel? *I said out of the cloud.* She just smiled and said, good, huh? I was so happy. Ok, do it again! This time she put buzzers into my hands and a headset that was clicking. I did not know what to expect, but I was so excited as I had not felt like this for 20 years. I cried a lot, again.

The next day, I suffered badly again and messaged her that I was really sorry, but I am not coming back as it's too much, I can't deal with it. But the same as the first time, on the fifth day, I was begging her to book me in again.

I cried, and I was emotional as I realised that this is working. I would love to experience it again with more awareness, as I was not sure what was happening. I had a few sessions with her, and it was the best thing I could have done to recover.

It felt like the Matrix tbh. It was fantastic to see what my own brain was doing for me, and I started to function again, and I was the happiest person you can imagine. The therapy was such a benefit to my mental health, like nothing I had experienced before.

To sleep again, smile and laugh, and be excited about things and function normally again is great. We don't appreciate it enough, as we are so used to it. We exhaust ourselves for others, for companies, to feel good, maybe? Or keep busy, so we don't have to face problems that we have bottled up.

Along with many other people who have gone through break downs, burn outs and reached rock bottom, I have to say that this was one of the best things that happened to me in my life.

It was probably the hardest challenge I have had to face, but it taught me so much about self-care and opened my eyes so much that if I live from now on being aware of and looking after my mental health, maybe my best years are ahead of me. I cut all the toxic people from my life, I sleep more than I ever did, and I love how much I can enjoy things that I never appreciated before.

I learnt to put myself first, and looking after myself is my priority.

It never was before.

I had a moment while going through the recovery where I was brushing my teeth, and I was not able to look at myself in the mirror, as I was ashamed of what I did to myself.

I nearly let those nasty people eat me alive, I let myself get so low, I nearly died as I wanted to be that good person. It was an odd moment, as I felt like I had helped others not to fall, but not myself!

I will die another day. When my time is up … not yet.

Things are much better now, and I use emdr on my phone app about once a month as I believe it should be mandatory for anyone going through stress. The best thing is no pills, no talking, just me and my brain. Sometimes I use it just to clear my brain. I sleep really well after this.

There are YouTube videos where you can just watch the screen and switch off. There are many ways therapists use it. It can be either clicks, lights, vibrations or moving a ball on the screen.

We were born mentally healthy. What happened to us, and our bad coping mechanisms created problems for us. Body can recover after trauma. Brain has a capability too, and EMDR helped me a lot with that.

About EMDR therapy

I was so fascinated by this therapy I was curious to find out as much as I could. I also knew how many people could benefit from it. I was amazed it's my own body that is healing me.

This therapy is called Eye Movement Desensitization and Reprocessing (EMDR). Many people that suffer from complex PTSD, PTSD, anxiety, panic attacks, addictions, emotional traumas, depression can benefit from this.

To describe it, you go back to situations that caused you distress, but it feels like a movie you are watching, but you feel safe, and you process it differently.

It was fascinating.

Your body takes you there through feelings, but you are safe, and you see it differently. If you've seen the Matrix, I would describe it like this, but in real life, as I don't actually know how to describe it, only as something totally fascinating.

Another amazing thing is that it's fast! After three sessions, I felt very different. I loved it. The whole experience was fascinating. Very painful, but also beautiful. I have no other words for it.

The other great benefit is you don't need to talk to a person. If you don't want to talk about it, you don't, and the therapist takes you through it. No one needs to know your traumas if you don't want to.

Isn't it amazing?

Research shows that eye movement in REM sleep is very similar to EMDR eye movement. The more REM sleep we get, the less likely we are to become depressed.

PTSD is notoriously associated with disturbed sleep, and self-medication with drugs or alcohol further disrupts REM sleep.

By taking drugs, you can numb the feelings and events, as they can blunt the images and sensations of terror, but they remain embedded in the mind and body. But research shows that those who received EMDR no longer experience the distinct imprints of the trauma.

It just becomes the story of the event.

It's the story that no longer matters and no longer affects you.

Quiz: How do you feel today?

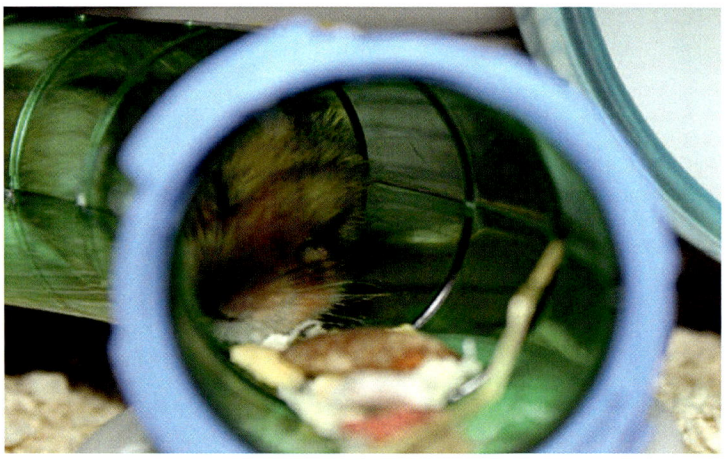

A) Stuck in the hole

B) Safe in the hole

C) Can't get out of the hole

D) Happy in the hole

Chapter 9

FOOD EVERYWHERE

MY WEEK OF CLEAN EATING

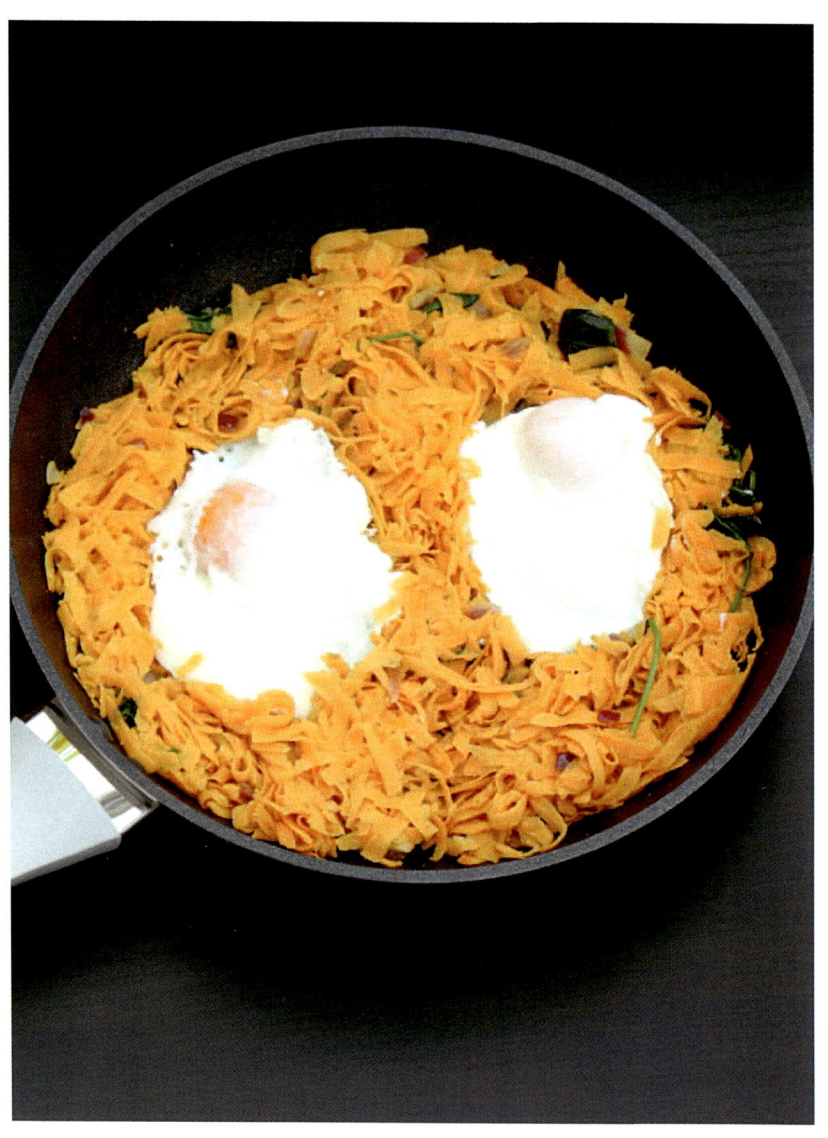

DRINKS

I am going to repeat myself here a little as I really would like you to understand it, so it becomes simple for you: Knowledge is the Key.

I hope that many of you will stop overcomplicating it as much as many do.

Every morning I have a cup of coffee, as I really like to start my morning with a fresh cup. Some days I have freshly squeezed orange juice, but I am just going to focus on food. If you do like to have fresh juice every morning, I definitely recommend it.

Fresh juice: If you like to have an orange juice, that is great, but keep in mind it must be freshly squeezed. No box juice, no bought juice, as we want to make sure we are in control of what exactly is in it. Only oranges, lemons, limes, or any other fruits you like freshly squeezed at home.

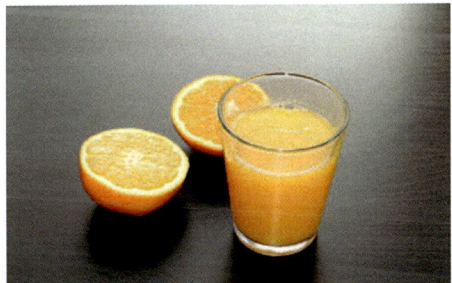

If you are one of those people that don't function in the morning without coffee, I have good news for you. One coffee a day is good for you, as it wakes your body up and speeds everything up a little. If with milk, full fat or half fat organic milk.

The bad news is, that you can only have one coffee a day for your week of clean eating. More than one coffee a day has a bad effect on the insulin response in your body.

I am not great with drinking water, so what I do, I make myself a cup of mint tea (my favourite) or any other tea when I get bored of mint and add a spoonful of honey or maple syrup.

You should have 8 glasses of water, so either you drink tea or water, it's up to you.

If you don't like pure water, you can put a jug of water into the fridge and put fruits, mint or lemon in and leave it to stand overnight. The next day you will have nice water with a fruity taste and full of vitamins.

Cashew milk

175-200 g of cashews

1liter of water

2 tbsp of honey or maple syrup

Vanilla extract (optional)

Salt and cinnamon (optional)

Soak the cashews overnight in water. Drain cashews and give them a good rinse. Add cashews into a blender, and add 1 litre of water. Add honey or maple syrup, vanilla extract, and blend everything together until milky and creamy.

Coffee

Should be with full fat milk. If you want a healthier option that is more clean and organic, you can make homemade almond milk, coconut milk or cashew milk.

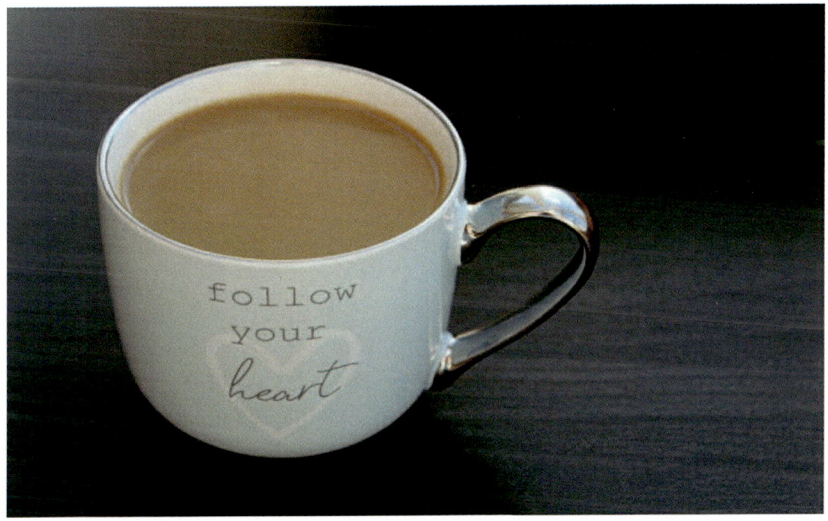

Monday Breakfast

EGGS, VEG, RADDISH

Can either have scrambled eggs with veg together or cook separately. If there is any veg, you don't like, simply replace it with veg you like.

Remember, to send your metabolism to work, so it does not go into sleep mode is to eat within an hour after waking up. Even if it means a handful of peanuts or a spoonful of peanut butter.

Ingredients

2 Eggs

Radish or tomato as you wish

Handful of organic spinach

Pine nuts to sprinkle

Red onion

Garlic

Mushrooms

Salt, Pepper

Spoonful of coconut fat or olive oil

Place one spoonful of coconut fat in a pan and bring it to a medium heat. Add onion, garlic and stir for a few minutes. Add spinach and mushrooms, salt and pepper, stir for a few minutes and sprinkle with pine nuts.

Put on the side of the plate or use a different pan and bring it to a medium heat. Add a spoonful of coconut fat (olive oil or butter) and break two eggs. Stir until ready to serve.

Wash and cut radish into halves.

Coconut fat: Oil for your metabolism to work, pine nuts, spinach, and other veg as nutrients for your well-being and health.

Enjoy.

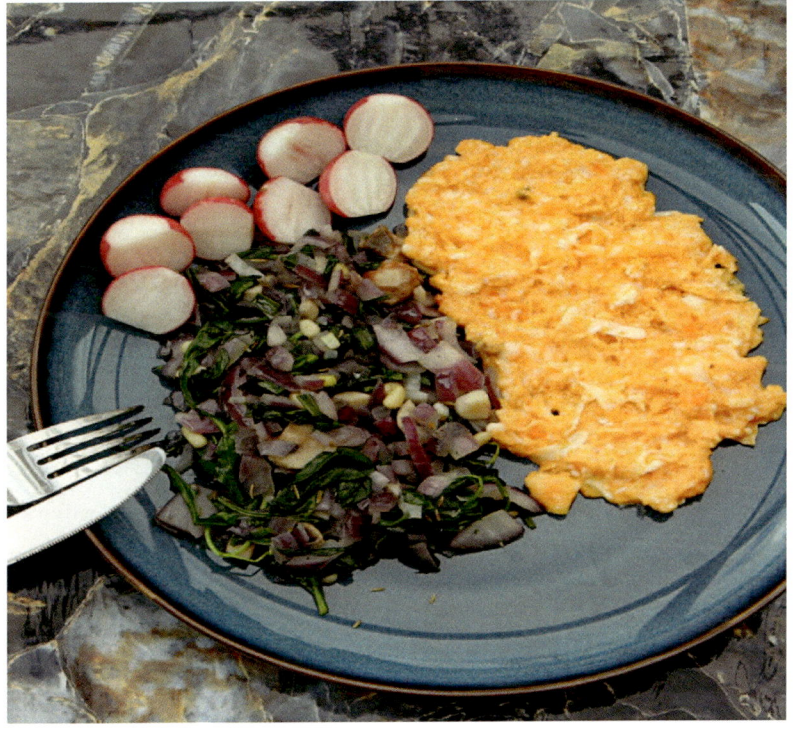

This dish is approximately 230 calories.

Monday Lunch

STIR FRY SEA BASS

Ingredients

Sea bass fillet

Cabbage

Edamame beans

Baby corn

Pepper

Onion

Asparagus

Garlic

Pomegranate seeds

Pine nuts

Lime juice

Heat the olive oil in a frying pan over a medium to high heat. Season the sea bass with salt and pepper, and when the oil is hot, lay the fish skin side down in the pan.

Cook without turning for 2-3 minutes, then flip it over. Remove the heat and let the fish finish cooking in residual heat.

Heat a wok or saucepan on high heat and add olive oil or butter. Add cabbage, beans, asparagus (precooked), onion, pepper, baby corn, garlic and stir fry for 2 minutes. I added a spoonful of pesto, salt and pepper and a tablespoonful of water. Stir for another 2 minutes or until the vegetables are cooked (on my normal week, I add spoon of soy sauce instead of pesto).

Place vegetables on the dish, sprinkle with pomegranate and pine nuts and place the sea bass over the vegetables. Add lime juice and parsley.

Enjoy.

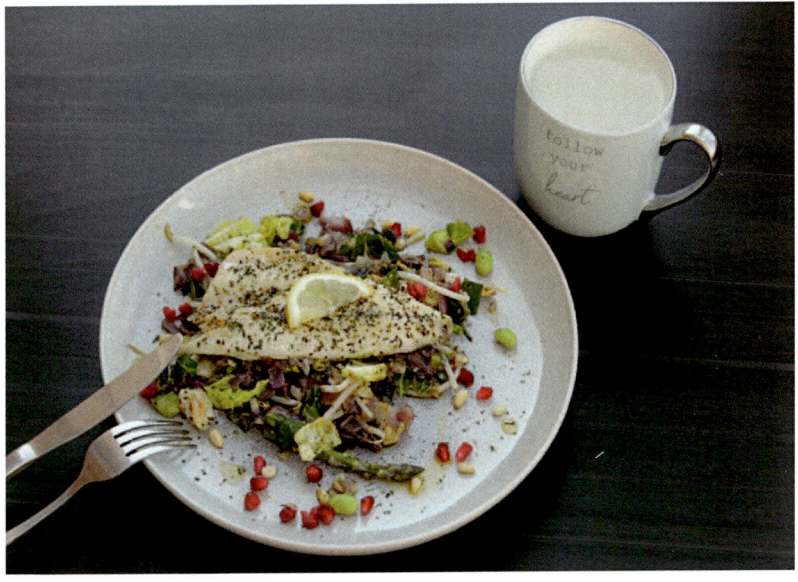

This dish is approximately 300 calories.

Monday Dinner

OVEN BAKED VEG

Ingredients

Brussel sprouts

Baby sweetcorn

Red onion

Butternut squash

Chilli, Garlic

Cooked broccoli

Red and yellow peppers

Courgette

Carrot

Cut all vegetables into chunks and place into a bowl.

Mix and add olive oil, add salt and pepper and spread evenly on a baking tray and roast for 15 minutes and stir. Roast for another 10 minutes or until veg is crispy.

Optional: (for people with sweet taste preferences) Mix olive oil, honey, lime juice, salt and pepper and mix together with veg. Place onto baking tray and place into the oven.

For this dish, you can add any root vegetables you like, such as parsnip, celeriac, asparagus.

Enjoy.

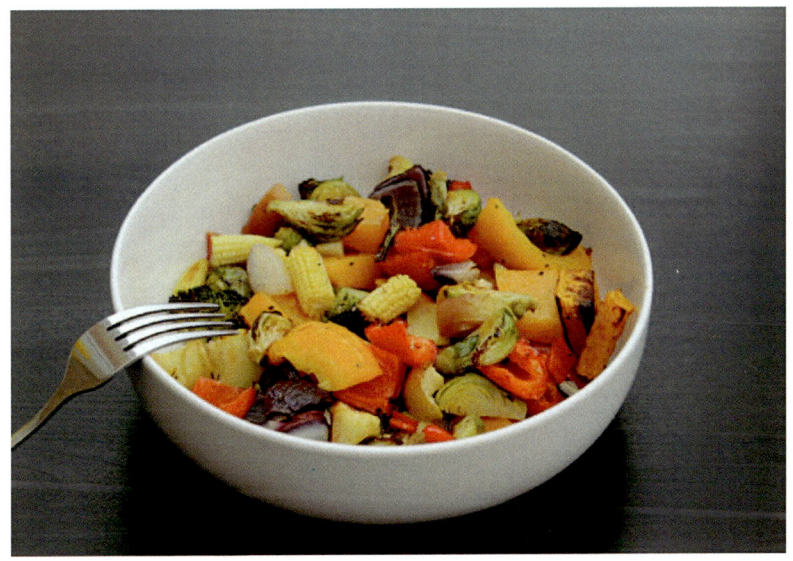

This dish is approximately 300 calories.

Snack in the morning

Handful of blueberries

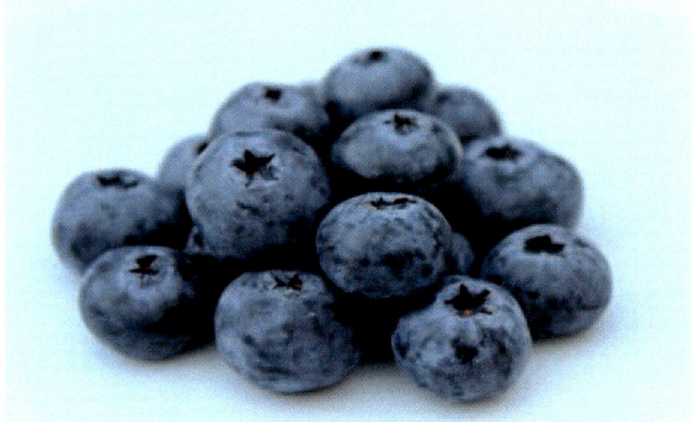

Approximately 50 calories

Snack in the evening

Handful of walnuts and dried papaya and pineapple.

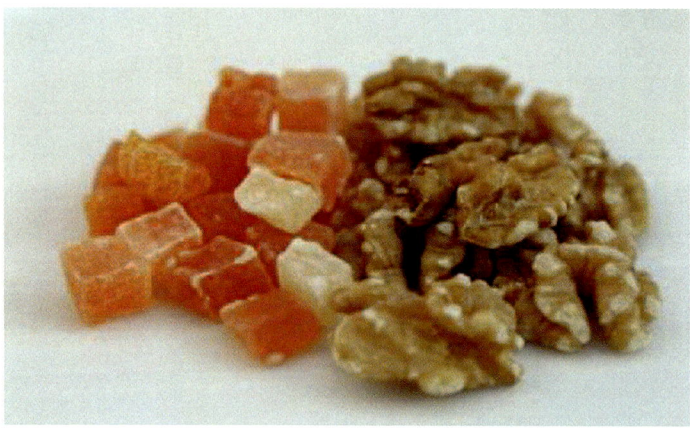

Approximately 150 calories

I had another two large mugs of tea (pint size). I added a spoonful of honey into each of them, and before the bed, I am having another tea.

I had mint tea, strawberry and lime tea and chamomile tea before bed. I also had a glass of water and a cup of coffee.

If you want to calculate my income of calories with honey, you would get to around 1,150 calories on Monday. It means I am possibly going to be hungry. In this case what I do is have another handful of my snack blueberries and later on possibly a handful of walnuts or some other healthy snack such as a few pieces of ham or whatever I find 'clean' in the fridge. These calories are much easier for the body to process, and it's healthy. It depends on what you want to do. If you are losing weight, you can calculate your formula, which I showed you in an earlier chapter, keep the deficit of 500 calories there, or keep your daily income and keep the weight on.

I don't calculate calories. I just eat more good than bad, and If I feel like I have put weight on, I go cleaner for a few days and return to my original weight. But I have been the same weight for years.

My insulin stays in balance as there is no heavily processed food.

Tuesday Breakfast

CARROT, APPLE, PEANUT BUTTER DISH

Ingredients

2 Carrots

1 Apple

Spoonful of mixed seeds

Coconut flakes

Spoonful of peanut butter

Maple syrup

Walnuts

Optional: Add small banana, cocoa peanut butter

Heat the coconut oil in the pan on a medium heat. Add grated carrots, apple, spoonful of seeds, walnuts, and stir for about 2-3 minutes.

Place on the dish, sprinkle with coconut flakes, add spoonful of peanut butter and maple syrup or honey according to your preference.

Enjoy.

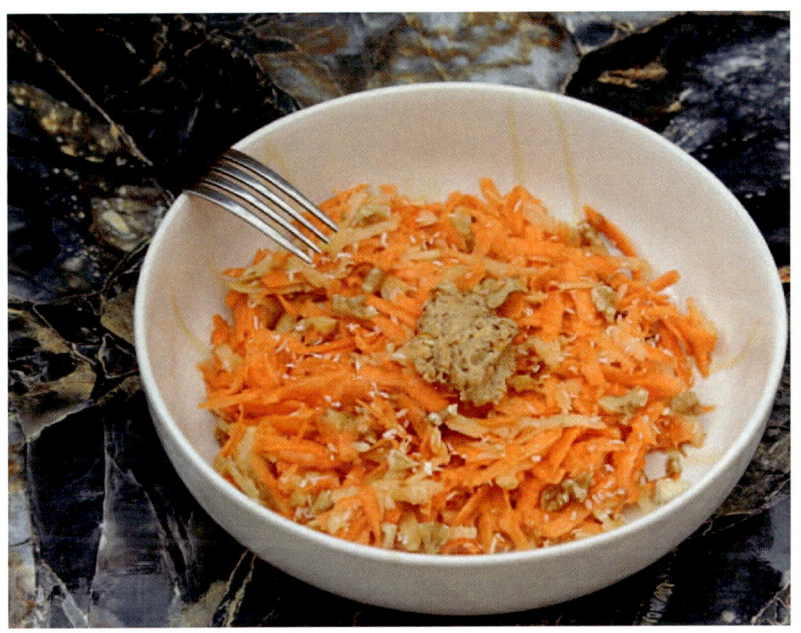

Average 350 calories

Tuesday Lunch

CHICKEN SALAD

Ingredients

2 Chicken breasts

Red and yellow peppers

Sweetcorn

Red onion, Spring onions

Avocado

Tomatoes

Olive oil, Lime juice

Coriander

Salt, Pepper

Garlic

Melt the coconut oil in a large saucepan on a medium heat. Add onion, garlic and chicken cut into small pieces, salt, pepper, and cook for 3-4 minutes.

Chop remaining ingredients into bite size pieces.

Add chicken mixture to vegetables in a bowl.

Season with a dressing of olive oil and lime juice.

Add coriander leaves to garnish.

Enjoy.

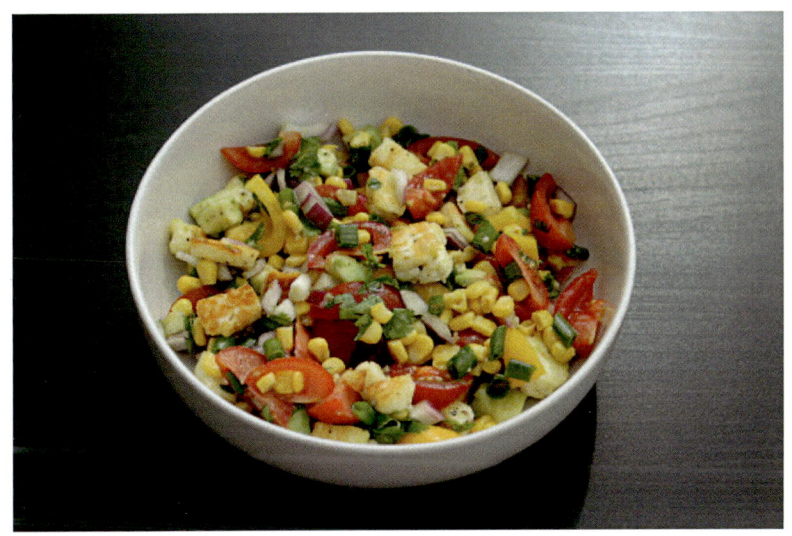

Approximately 360 calories.

Tuesday Dinner

PLANTAIN CURRY

Ingredients

1 Tbsp Coconut oil (or any kind of cold pressed oil you use)

2 Shallots, finely chopped

2 Cloves garlic, finely chopped

1 Red pepper

1 Red chilli

1 Tsp Cinnamon

2 Tsp Cumin powder

¼ Tsp Nutmeg

3 Plantains, sliced

200g Chickpeas (pre - cooked)

200ml Homemade veg stock

6 Large tomatoes

4 Sprigs fresh thyme, finely chopped (or use seasoning)

1 Juice of lime

Salt and pepper

Place 1 tbsp of coconut oil into a large pot on a medium heat. Add the shallots, garlic, salt, pepper, cumin, nutmeg, cinnamon and stir slightly, then allow to simmer for 2 minutes.

Add thyme, peppers, chopped tomatoes. Stir in the other ingredients and allow to cook for 5 minutes.

Pour in stock, chickpeas, sliced chilli and the juice of a lime. Simmer over a medium heat for 10-15 minutes.

Optional: You can add plantain whilst you are adding tomatoes into a bowl or use the oven. (I prefer the oven)

Plantain: heat the oven to a high temperature, 420 degrees. Cut plantain into chips, place on baking paper, sprinkle with salt, pepper and drizzle with olive oil (coconut fat can be used). After 10 minutes, flip them over and cook for another 10 minutes, until golden and crispy.

Optional: I added to my curry, mushrooms, spinach, asparagus, baby sweetcorn. Can add sweet potato if you wish. You could also use bananas instead of plantain.

In any recipes, if I have used anything, you don't like, simply replace them with something different or do not use the ingredient.

Enjoy.

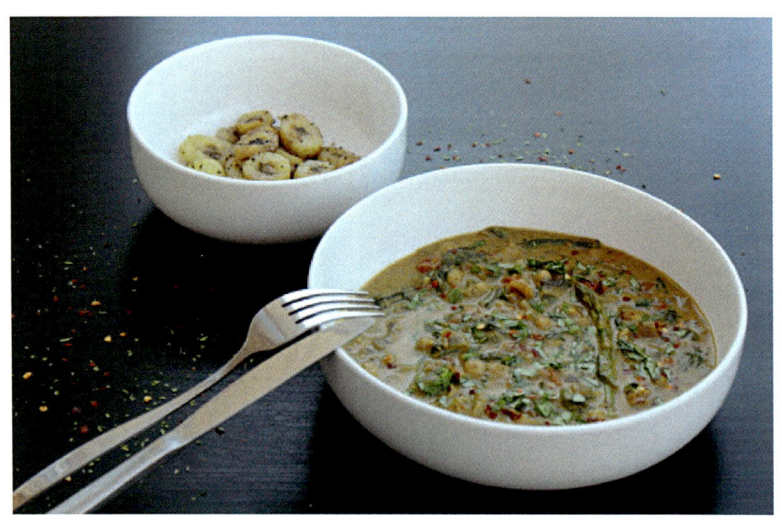

(Adapted from runningonrealfood.com)

Approximately 400 calories

Snack in the morning

An apple

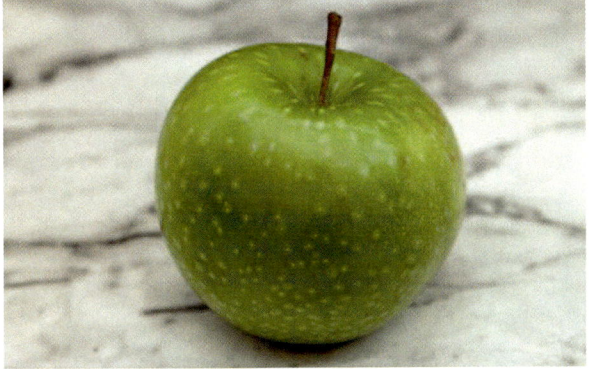

Approximately 50 calories

Snack in the evening

Handful of pistachios

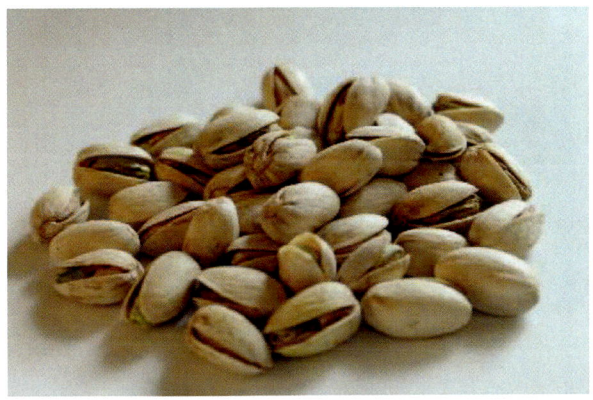

Approximately 70 calories

1 coffee, 3 large fruit teas (honey or maple syrup), glass of water.

Approximately daily income of calories 1,350.

Wednesday Breakfast

GREEK YOGHURT, STRAWBERRIES, BANANA

Ingredients

100-150 g of full fat organic Greek yoghurt

2 Strawberries

1 Small banana

6 Pecans

6 Blueberries

Coconut flakes

Maple syrup or honey

Optional: cinnamon, spoon of peanut butter

Place organic yoghurt into a bowl and add remaining ingredients.

Sprinkle with coconut flakes and add spoonful of maple syrup or honey if desired.

If you can't go completely organic, then at least try to buy the following organic due to high levels of pesticides and chemicals: Strawberries, kale, spinach, apples, grapes, nectarines, peaches, cherries, pears, tomatoes, celery.

Enjoy.

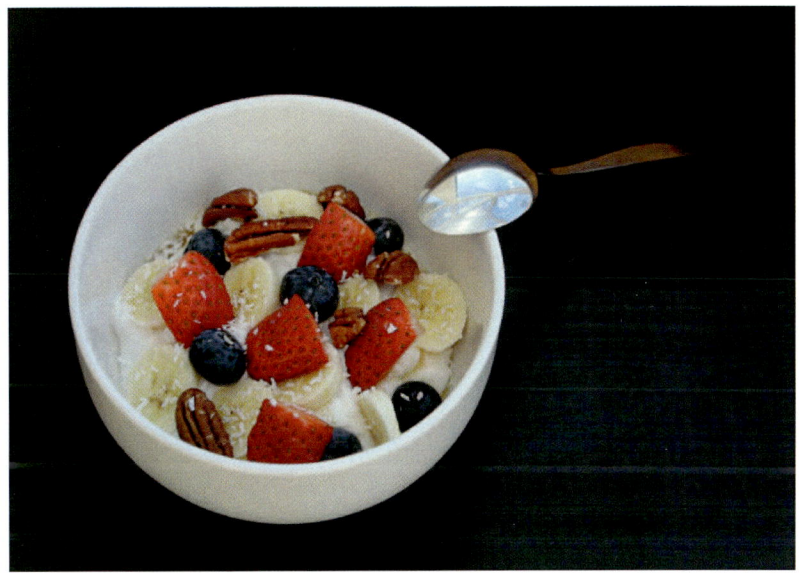

Approximately 350 calories

Wednesday Lunch

SALMON WITH SWEET POTATO FRIES

Ingredients

Onion, Garlic

Pine nuts

Cherry tomatoes

Mixed salad

Asparagus

Sweet potato

Salmon fillet

Mushrooms

Cinnamon

Salt, Pepper

Seasoning

Lemon

Peel and cut sweet potato to slices. Place onto baking paper, add cumin salt, pepper and olive oil. Place into preheated oven 180 degrees. Bake for 10 minutes and turn around. Add cinnamon and bake for another 10-15 minutes until cooked.

Meanwhile fries in the oven heat a pan on medium heat with olive oil and add onion, garlic and salad and stir for 3-4 minutes. Add pine nuts and tomatoes and stir for another 2 minutes. You can add mushrooms or fry them separately in butter and smashed garlic for 3-4 minutes until slightly brown.

Place asparagus into a pot and after boiling, cook for another 2 minutes.

Sprinkle salmon fillet with salt and pepper. Place olive oil into a pan and heat up on medium for around 2 minutes. Add heat to medium-high. Place salmon on its skin into the pan and press on fish for around 10 seconds. Reduce heat to medium until skin is crispy, about 5-6 minutes. Carefully turn the salmon over and press for 10 seconds. And cook for another 2-3 minutes. Place onto a plate.

Sauce for salmon: Heat olive oil or butter, add 1 table spoonful of minced garlic and 1 spoonful of lemon zest, stir for 30 seconds. Add lemon juice, salt and black pepper. Stir and cook for 1 minute.

Enjoy. (400 calories)

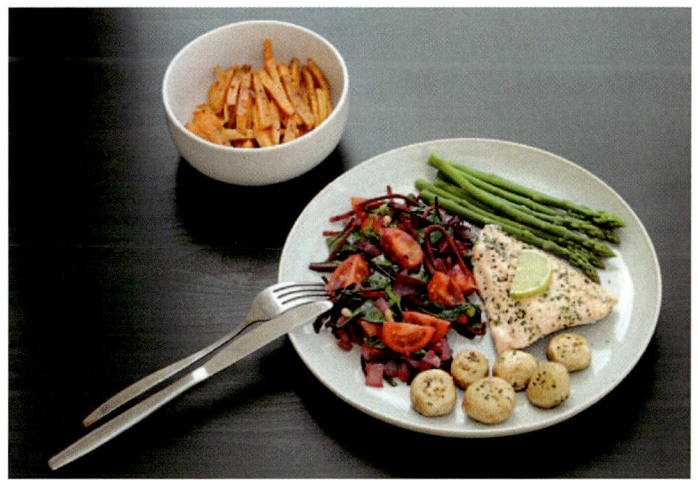

Wednesday Dinner

BAKED BROCOLLI AND CAULIFLOWER

Ingredients

Broccoli

Cauliflower

Spring onion

Cashews

Cheese

Butter

Milk

Onions

Garlic

Preheat the oven to 220C. Cook the cauliflower and broccoli in boiling water for 5-6 minutes until tender.

Cut into small pieces garlic and onion and place into a baking dish with spoonful of butter.

Drain vegetables and tip into baking dish.

Heat the milk and butter in a saucepan over medium heat, whisking constantly. Reduce the heat and add grated cheddar, salt and pepper, and on very low heat whisk until cheese melting.

Add cashews into a dish and pour the sauce over broccoli and cauliflower. Bake for 20 minutes or until the top is golden. Sprinkle with spring onions.

Enjoy.

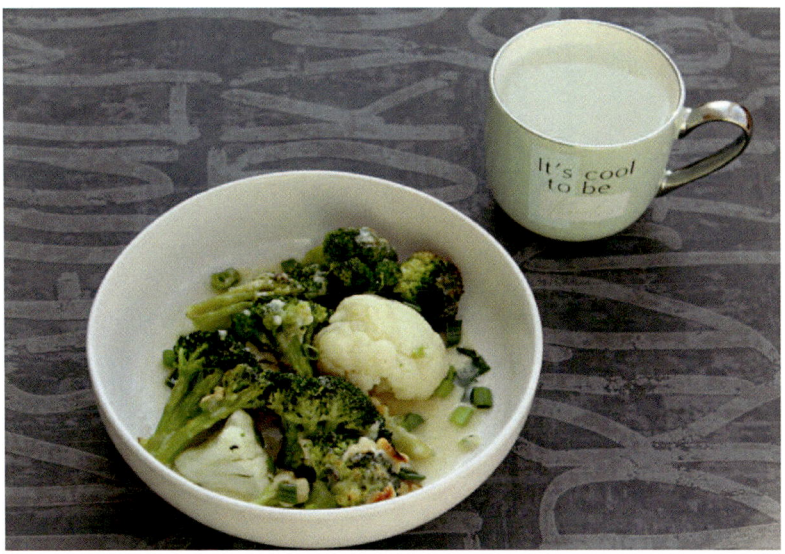

This dish is Approximately 150 calories

Snack in the morning

Pomegranate seeds

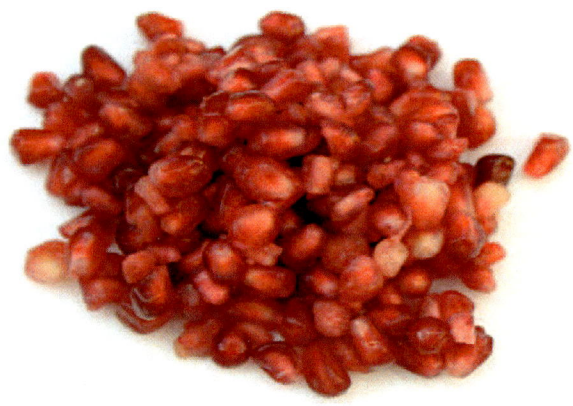

Approximately 85 calories

Snack in the evening

Half of avocado

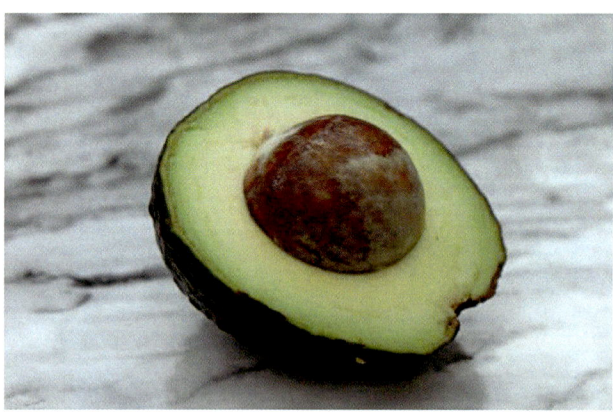

Approximately 130 calories

This daily income comes to around 1,250 calories a day. Again, it's low. It's healthy. You can add a snack or if you get hungry in the evening, have half a banana. See how you feel. If you are in your first 3 days, you will definitely be hungry.

Thursday Breakfast

SMOOTHIE

Ingredients

Milk, Maple syrup or honey

Banana

Peanut butter

Salt

Place milk, banana, add a pinch of salt, spoonful of maple syrup and peanut butter into a blender and blend until smooth.

You can use any fruits or veg you like for your smoothies. The choice is yours.

For my smoothies, I use Meridian coconut and peanut butter or Meridian cocoa and peanut butter, if you fancy a chocolate taste.

Enjoy.

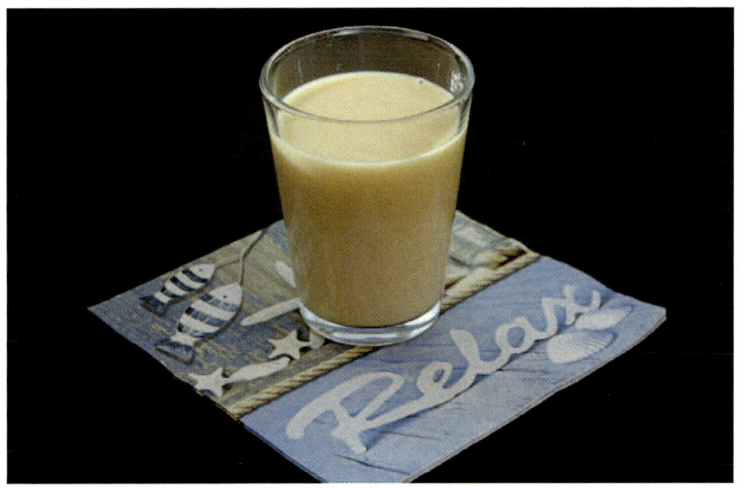

Approximately 220 calories

Thursday Lunch

KIDNEY BEAN CURRY

Ingredients

1 Tbsp Olive oil

1 Onion freshly chopped

2 Garlic cloves, freshly chopped

Thumb-size piece of ginger, peeled and finely chopped, leaves roughly shredded

Coriander finely chopped

1 Tsp Ground cumin

1 Tsp Paprika

2 Tsp Garam masala

400 g Freshly chopped cherry tomatoes

400 g Kidney beans precooked

Salt, Pepper

Heat the olive oil in a large frying pan over a low-medium heat. Add the onion and pinch of salt and stir occasionally. Add the garlic, coriander, and ginger and cook for another 2-3 minutes until fragrant.

Add the spices to the pan and cook for another 1-2 mins. Tip tomatoes and kidney beans into a pan and little bit of water if needed. Bring to boil.

Turn down the heat and simmer for 15 minutes until the curry is nice and thick. Season to taste, then serve and add coriander leaves.

Optional: you can add chilli

Enjoy.

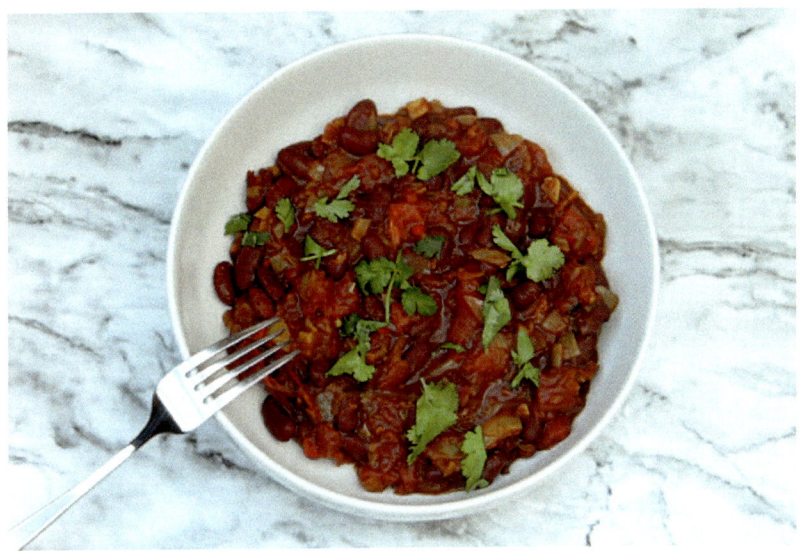

This dish is Approximately 270 calories

Thursday Dinner

SPICY AFRICAN PEANUT STEW WITH CELERIAC FRIES

Ingredients

2 Onions

2 Gloves of garlic

1 ½ a Thumb size piece of ginger

1 Fresh red chilly

450 g of Chickpeas (prepared)

250g Oyster mushrooms

2 Sweet potato

¼ of a Head of white cabbage

1 ½ Tsp of salt

Homemade veg stock (or use seasoning)

1 Tbsp Ground cumin

1 Tbsp Ground coriander

1 Tbsp Sweet paprika

125g Peanut butter

2 Tomatoes chopped

100g Baby spinach

Juice of 1 lime

Homemade veg stock: 2 celery sticks, 1 carrot, 1 onion, 1-2 garlic cloves, 5 peppercorns, 1 leek, salt, spoonful of olive oil. Heat oil in a soup pot, add chopped vegetables and cook for 5-10 mins, add water and salt and on low temperature cook for another 30 mins. Strain and discard vegetables.

Reason for a homemade veg stock is for this week, we try to go as clean as possible and you can keep the stock in the fridge for up to 2 weeks; stock bought in a supermarket can be used for up to 2 years! The same for the chickpeas.

Peel and dice the onions, garlic and ginger, mushrooms, sweet potatoes (leave the skin or peel as you wish), cut the cabbage into long thin strips. Slice the chilli.

Heat a large non-stick pan on high heat. Once hot, add onions, garlic, chilli, mushrooms and fry for 5 mins, stirring regularly to prevent them sticking. If they start to stick, add a teaspoonful of water and stir to loosen.

Once the onions have started to brown, add the chopped sweet potatoes and cabbage, a pinch of salt and add 50ml of homemade veg stock. Stir, put the lid on and allow to cook for another 10-15 mins, until the sweet potato starts to soften. Stir occasionally. Remove the lid, add the ground cumin., coriander and paprika and mix well.

Put the remaining veg stock and add (ideally organic) peanut butter into a jug and mix so that it starts to combine. Pour this sauce over the cooked veg, add chopped tomatoes, bring to boil, then reduce to a simmer for 5 mins. Add the baby spinach and the lime juice. Taste and add seasoning as required. Salt, pepper and lime.

(the chickpeas and veg stock is ideally homemade for your clean eating. In this case, we used nearly all clean ingredients)

(in a normal week if you use organic veg stock and organic tinned chickpeas, you are still more than 80% clean ingredients)

CELERIAC FRIES

Heat the oven to 200 degrees. Cut the celeriac into fries and place on baking paper. Leave in the oven for 3-4 minutes and add olive oil or butter, cumin, salt and pepper.

Bake for about 10-15 minutes and then flip them over. Bake for another 15 minutes until the tops are nicely blistered.

Serve with a glass of water with lemon and mint.

Enjoy.

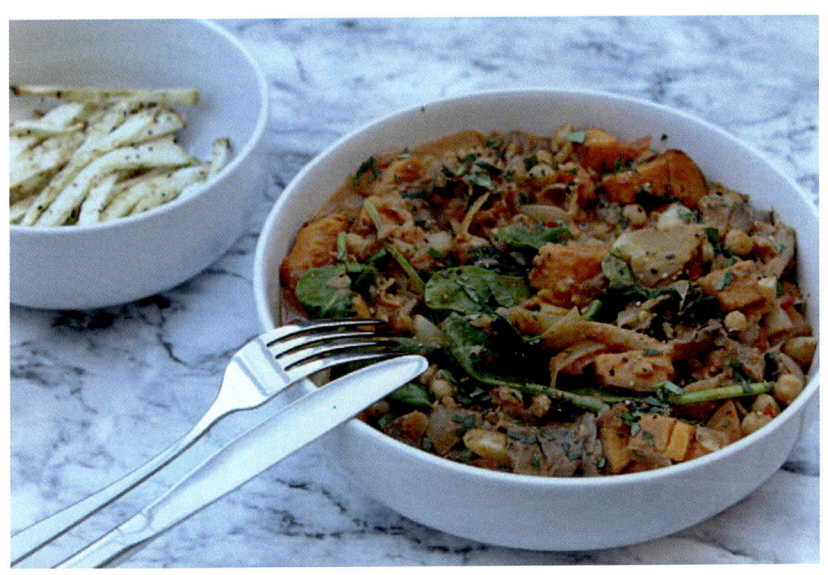

Dinner: Adapted by The Happy Health Plan (David & Stephen Flynn)

This dish is approximately 450 calories

Snack in the morning

Handful of cashews

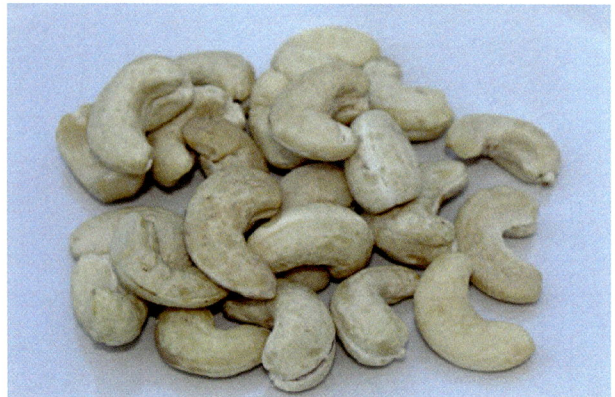

Approximately 100 calories (15-20 peanuts)

Snack in the evening

Carrots and hummus

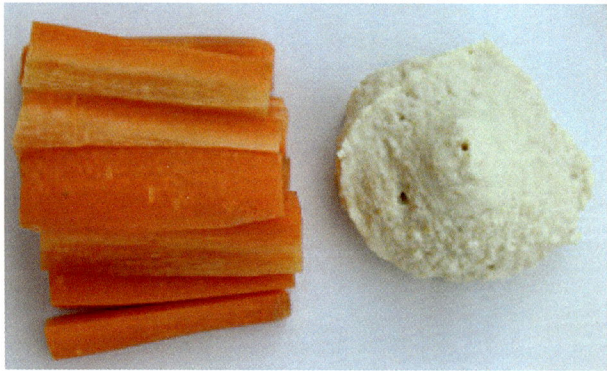

Approximately 100 calories

The daily income on Th is Approximately 1,200 calories. With a cup of coffee, 3 teas (2 one with a spoonful of honey and one with a spoonful of maple syrup, one plain) 2 glasses of water.

Friday Breakfast

SALAD WITH EGGS, OLIVES, TOMATOES

Ingredients

Cold salad

Olives

Grapes

Egg

Sesame oil

Cherry tomatoes

Walnuts

Half of avocado

Blue cheese

Seasoning

Salt

Pepper

Fill the pan with water, bring to boil, and add an egg. Boil for 7-8 minutes.

Meanwhile, wash cold salad and place into a bowl. Cut blue cheese and avocado into small pieces and add remaining ingredients into a bowl.

Shell and halve the egg, place it into the bowl.

Drizzle with olive oil or sesame oil up to your preferences and season with salt and pepper.

Enjoy.

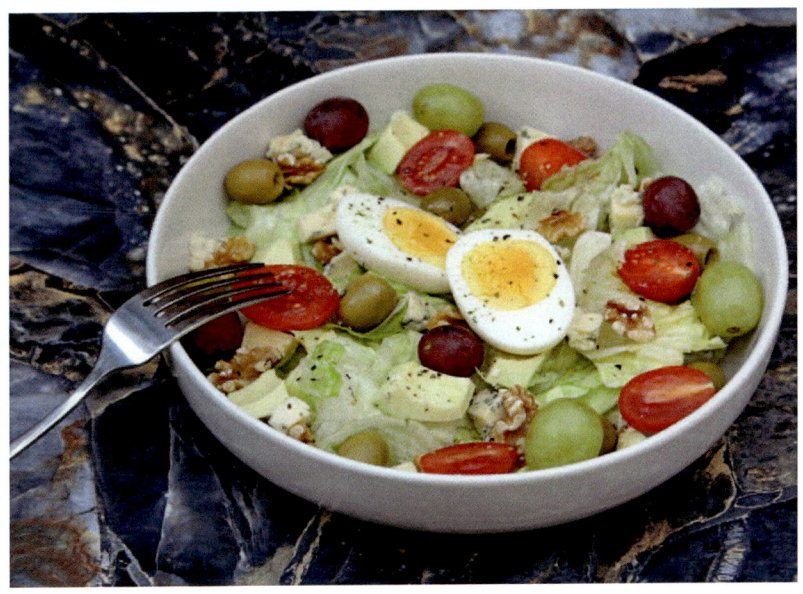

Approximately 430 calories.

Friday Lunch

THE GOODNESS BOWL

Ingredients

1 Onion

4 Tbsp Olive oil

1 Tbsp Maple syrup

4 Tbsp of Balsamic vinegar

200g Cherry tomatoes, 2 Tomatoes chopped

250g Lentils (precooked)

350g Butternut squash

1 Yellow and red pepper

1 Courgette

1 Avocado

2 Parsnips

100g Baby leaf spinach (organic)

Fresh flat-leaf parsley leaves

Salt, Pepper

Preheat oven to 180 degrees. Put 4 tablespoonfuls of olive oil, 4 tablespoonfuls of balsamic vinegar, maple syrup into a saucepan. Stir for 5 minutes, then add the lentils, stir through, remove from the heat and set aside.

Peel the squash, cut it in half and remove seeds. Cut into chunks. Tip into a roasting tray, drizzle with a little olive oil, season and roast in the oven for 15 mins, then remove.

Cut tomatoes, peppers, courgette, parsnips, butternut squash and add all cut vegetables to roasting tray, drizzle over a little more olive oil. Return to the oven to cook for another 15 minutes, until tender.

While the vegetables are roasting, halve the avocado and cut into small chunks. Wash and lightly chop the spinach and roughly chop the parsley leaves.

Remove the roasted veggies from the oven and tip into a serving bowl with the avocado, spinach, parsley and lentils.

(argument here whether balsamic vinegar is clean. We can easily replace canned food and veg stock, but it's harder to replace balsamic vinegar. You can either leave it out or accept 90% clean and use the balsamic vinegar. Enjoy. (450 cals)

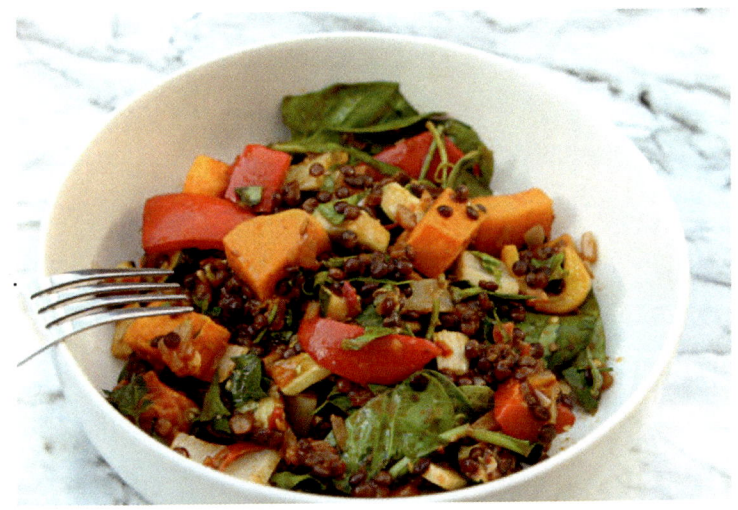

Friday Dinner

BUTTERNUT SQUASH SOUP

Ingredients

1 Butternut squash peeled and deseeded

Olive oil

1 Tbsp Butter

2 Onions

2 Mild red chillies

1 Garlic glove

750 ml Hot (for week of clean eating homemade) vegetable stock

Small cup of milk for a creamy taste, Coriander

Heat oven to 200C. Place peeled and cut butternut squash on large roasting tin with spoonful of olive oil.

Roast for 30 mins, turning once until soft.

While butternut placed in the oven, melt 1 tbsp butter with spoonful of olive oil in a large saucepan, add 2 diced onions, 1 sliced garlic and 2 deseeded and finally chopped red chillies.

Cover and cook on a low heat for 15 minutes until onions are soft.

Tip the butternut squash into the pan, add vegetable stock and a small cup of milk. Then whizz with a stick blender until smooth.

Return to the pan, gently reheat and season to taste. Enjoy.

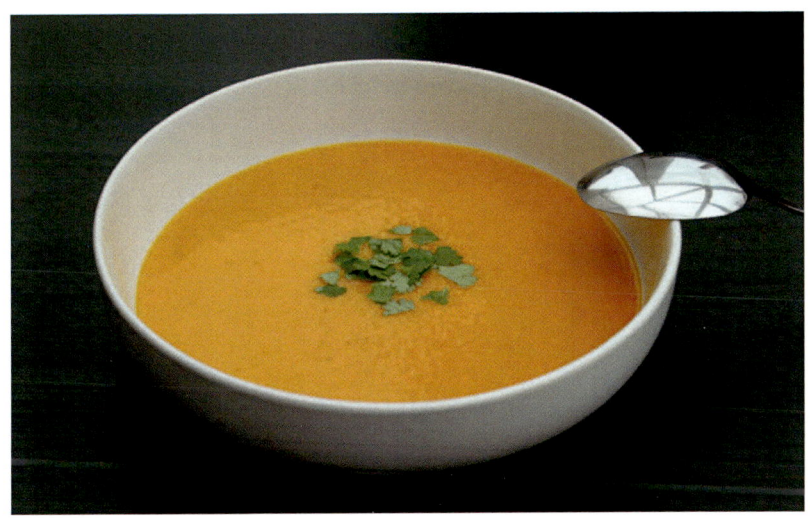

Approximately 150 calories

Snack in the morning

Kale crisps

Ingredients

Kale

Olive oil

Salt, Pepper

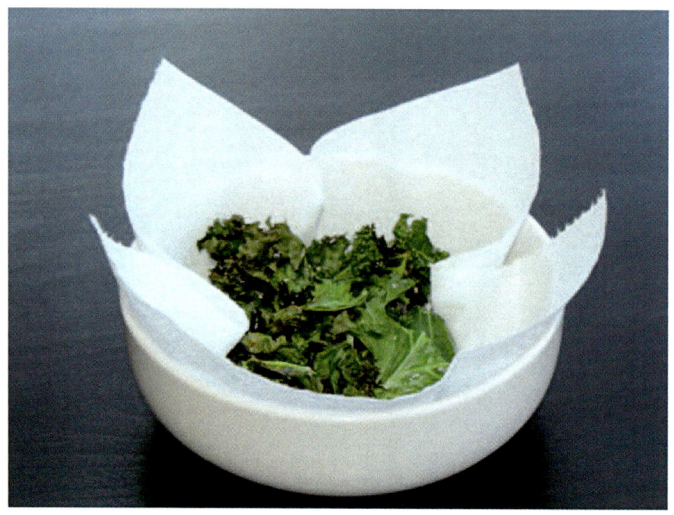

Approximately 100 calories

Heat the oven 150 C and place baking paper onto the tray. Wash the kale, cut into small pieces and place onto the baking paper. Drizzle with oil, sprinkle with salt and pepper and spread out in a single layer. Bake for 20 minutes or until crispy but still green.

Enjoy.

Snack in the afternoon

Small banana

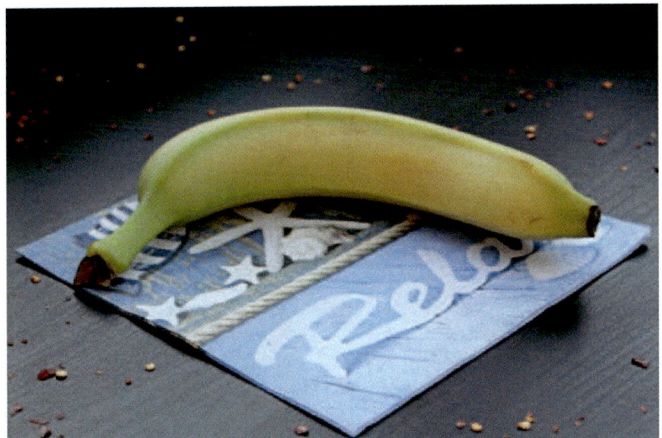

Approximately 90 calories.

The income of calories for Friday comes approximately to 1,350 calories.

Saturday Morning

PROSCIUTTO AND MELON SALAD

Ingredients

Rocket salad leaves

Melon

Parma ham

Pomegranate

Olive oil or rapeseed oil

Cut the melon into thick slices and remove the skin and seeds. Chop into chunks.

Place the melon around the plate and add parma ham and a freshly washed handful of rocket salad.

Season with black pepper, salt and drizzle with olive oil or rapeseed oil as you wish.

Enjoy.

Approximately 120 calories

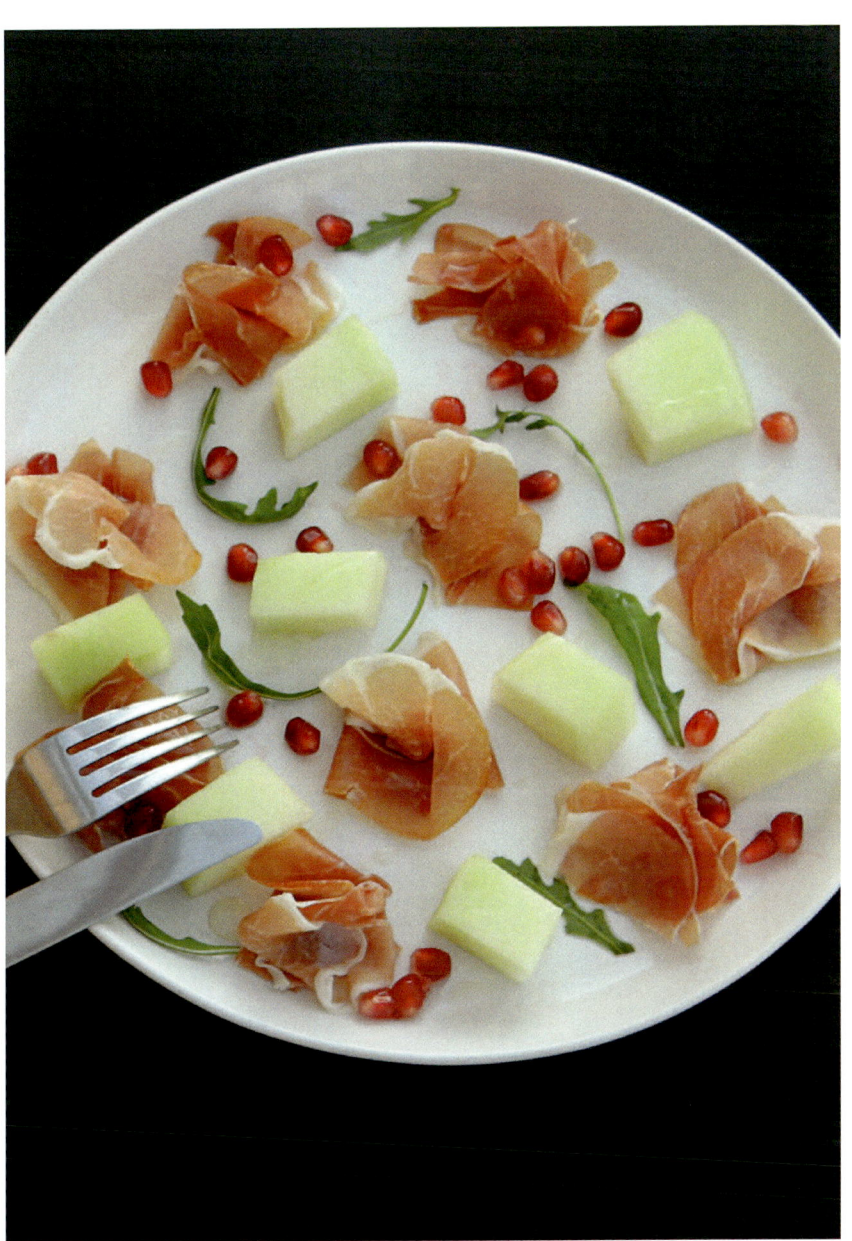

Saturday Lunch

BEEF STIR FRY

Ingredients

Carrot

Green cabbage

Beansprouts

White cabbage

Mixed pepper

Sweetcorn

Red onion

Beef

Salt

Pepper

Seasoning (Chinese 5 spice)

Beef marinade

Olive oil, Sesame oil or any cold pressed oil

Minced garlic

Fresh ginger

½ Tsp Chinese 5 spice (or spices you prefer)

Salt, Pepper

1 Tbs Honey

On your normal week, add 2 tbsp soy sauce, 1 tbsp red wine vinegar or white.

Combine marinade ingredients in bowl and add beef steak for 15 mins.

Heat cold pressed oil on medium high heat and place marinated steak on the pan and cook for 2-3 minutes, stirring to cook both sides. Remove the steak to a plate, leaving the marinade and oil in the pan.

Add 1 tbsp of sesame oil to the pan and add vegetables. Stir fry for another 4-5 minutes. Remove and add to the plate vegetables first. Place steak over the vegetables.

Enjoy.

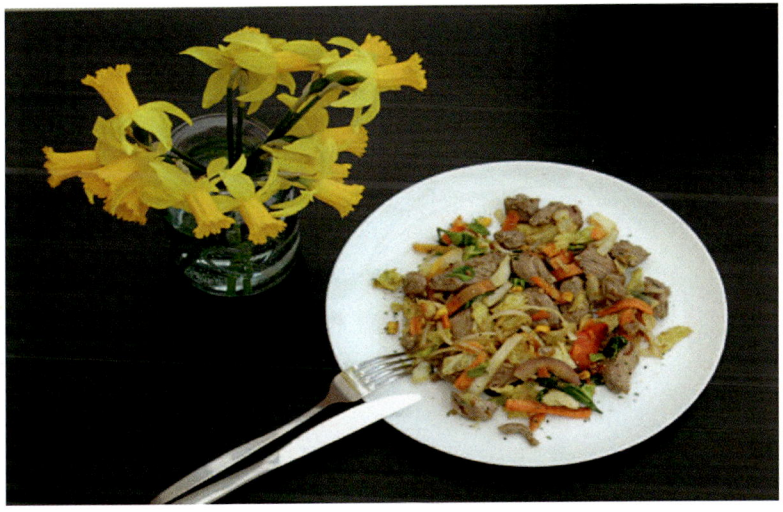

Approximately 300 calories

Saturday Dinner

ALOO GOBI

Ingredients

4 Spring onions

3 Garlic cloves

1 Fresh red chilli

½ Thumb sized piece of fresh ginger

1 to 2 Tbsp Coconut oil

1 Head of cauliflower

250g Broccoli florets

400ml Coconut milk

400ml Veg stock

2 Tbsp Tamari sauce

Seasoning

1 ½ Tbsp Black mustard seeds

1 Tbsp Ground turmeric

1 Tbsp Cumin seeds

1 Tsp Garam masala

Break cauliflower and broccoli into bite sized chunks, sprinkle on olive oil, and roast in pre-heated oven until soft and slightly charred.

Place some olive oil in a pan, add the garlic, spring onions, chilli and ginger and suate for a few minutes. Then add the roasted cauliflower and broccoli. Then add the spices and saute for a few more minutes.

Add the coconut milk, vegetable stock and tamari sauce and simmer for 20 minutes.

Season to taste and serve.

Enjoy.

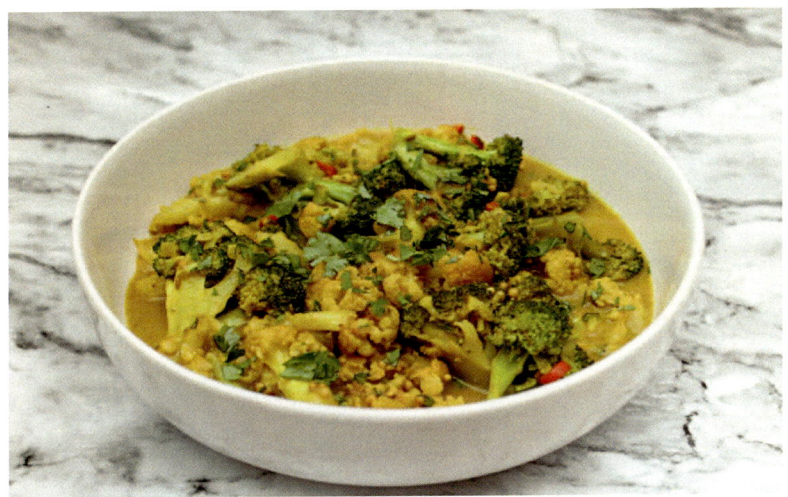

Approximately 300 calories

Adapted by The Happy Health Plan (David & Stephen Flynn)

Note: I replaced potato with broccoli, as broccoli is easier for metabolism than potato.

Saturday snack in the morning

Olives and feta cheese

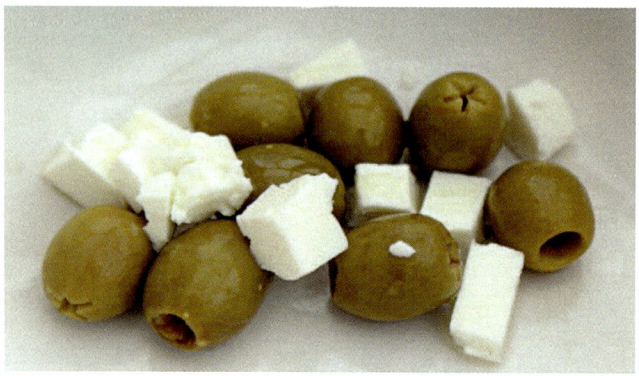

Approximately 120 calories

Saturday afternoon snack

Handful of mixed peanuts

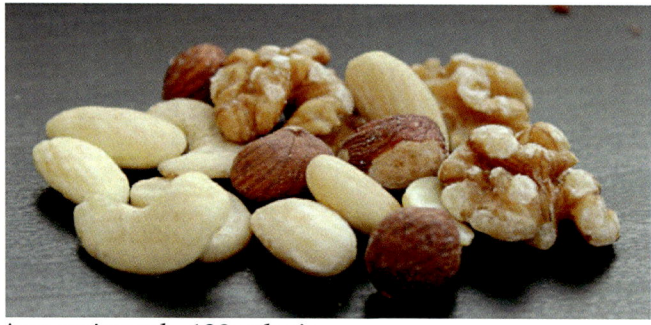

Approximately 120 calories

Saturday with drinks comes to Approximately 1,200 calories per day.

Sunday Breakfast

SWEET POTATO WITH EGGS AND SPINACH

You can also lay grated sweet potato, spinach, onion and garlic on the pan and stir for few minutes until soft. Whisk 2 eggs in the glass and pour over the potato and on small temperature let the egg cook. Sprinkle cheese and seasoning over the egg and potato and cook until soft.

Ingredients

1 Large sweet potato

2 Eggs

Spinach

Salt, Pepper

Coconut fat or organic unsalted butter

Onion

Garlic clove, minced

Thyme

Heat a spoonful of coconut fat in a large frying pan. Add finely cut onion, garlic and spinach leaves and cook on low to medium heat for 2-3 minutes. Add grated sweet potato salt, pepper and thyme and cook for another 3-4 minutes.

Meanwhile, heat water in a pan until the water simmers. Gently pour the eggs into hot water and cook for another 4 minutes on low heat.

Make 2 wells in the sweet potato and gently remove the eggs from the pan and place them into the holes. Cover and cook for another few minutes on low- medium heat (depending on how well you want the egg to be cooked).

Enjoy. (approx. 300 cals)

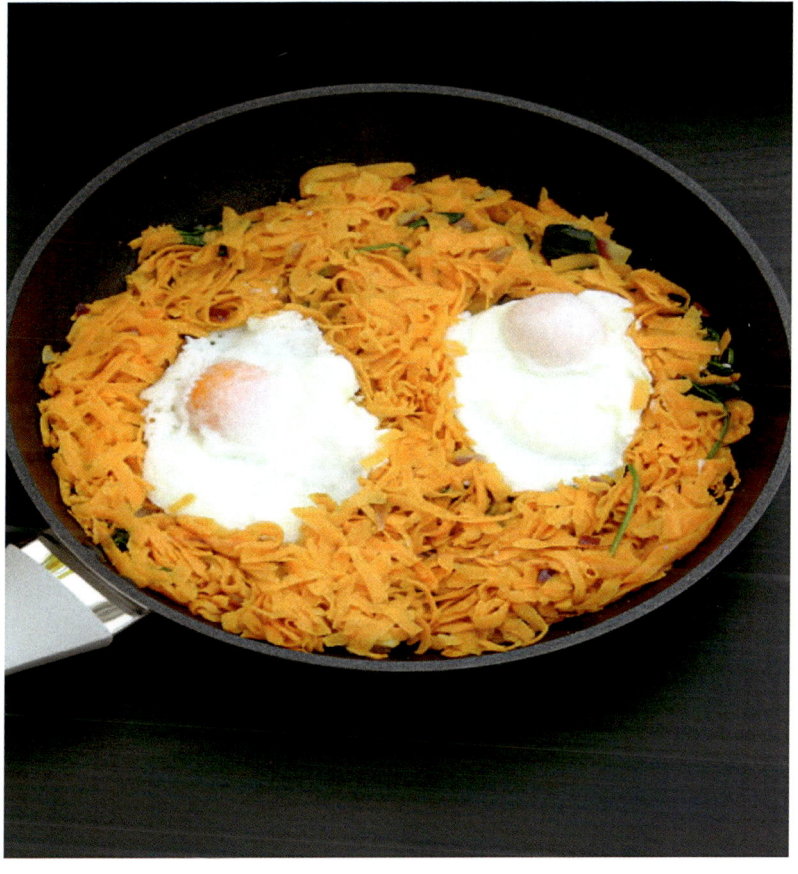

Sunday Lunch

ROASTED VEGETABLES WITH PEANUT SAUCE

Ingredients

Beetroot

Carrots

Parsnip

Onion

Spring onion

Unsalted roasted peanuts

Butternut squash

Seasoning

Ginger

Chilli

Salt

Pepper

Prepare all the veggies by slicing them lengthways.

Put 125g peanuts into blender, add 2 tbsp of water, 2 cm chopped piece of ginger root and ¼ of chilli, salt, pepper and blitz until smooth. If needed, add little bit of water or butter.

Place sliced veggies into a bowl and marinate for 5-10 minutes in the sauce, while preheating the oven to 180C.

Place marinated vegetables on baking paper and place in the oven for 20-30 minutes until the veggies are golden brown and cooked through. Drizzle with olive oil, top with freshly cut watercress and sprinkle with chopped spring onions. Season with salt and pepper.

On normal week I drizzle with Balsamic vinegar or add Tamari sauce to the peanut sauce.

Enjoy.

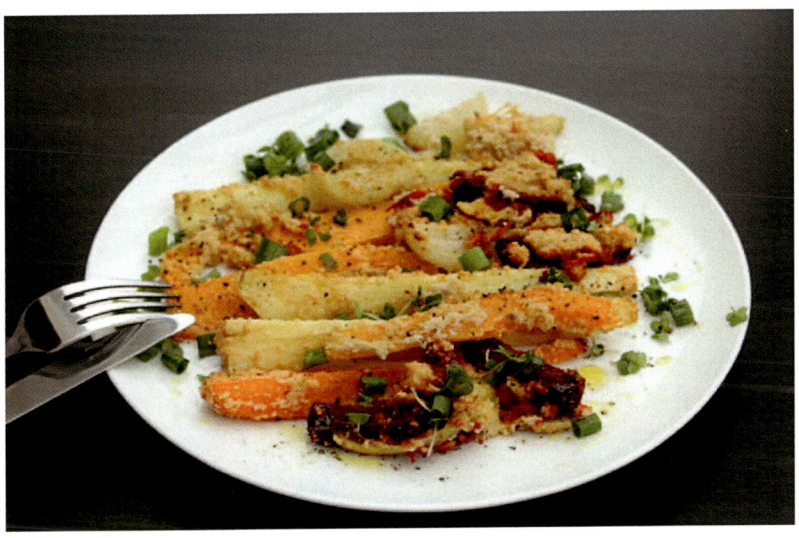

Approximately 400 calories

Sunday Dinner

TOMATO SALAD WITH MOZZARELLA

Ingredients

2 Large tomatoes

Organic full fat mozzarella

Olive oil

Seasoning

Salt

Pepper

Basil

(If you cannot find organic mozzarella, buy full fat mozzarella as full fat is less processed than half fat. On your normal week, you can use Balsamic vinegar for the flavour).

Cut two large tomatoes into chunks (optional cherry tomatoes) and place into a bowl.

Open and drain the bag of organic full fat mozzarella and cut into smaller pieces and mix well with the tomatoes.

Add salt and pepper, pour over about 1-2 tablespoons of olive oil. Cut fresh basil into small pieces and sprinkle over the dish.

Enjoy.

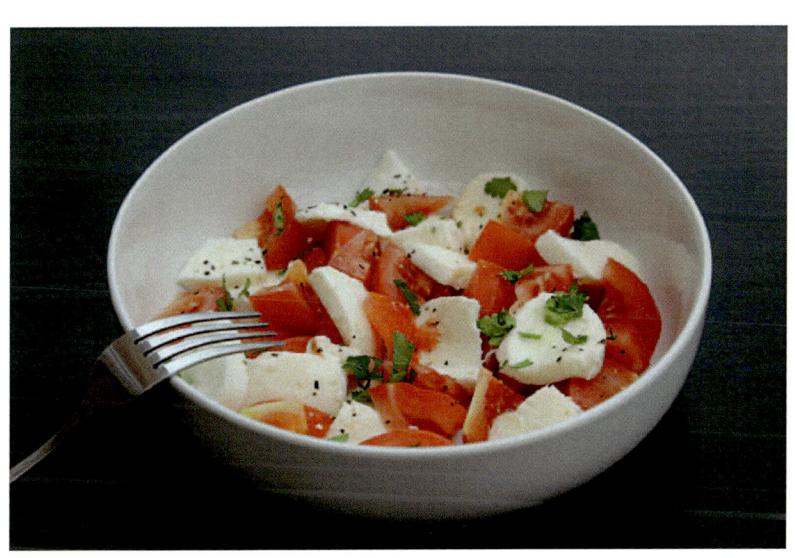

Approximately 280 calories

Snack in the morning

Handful of mixed fruit and nuts

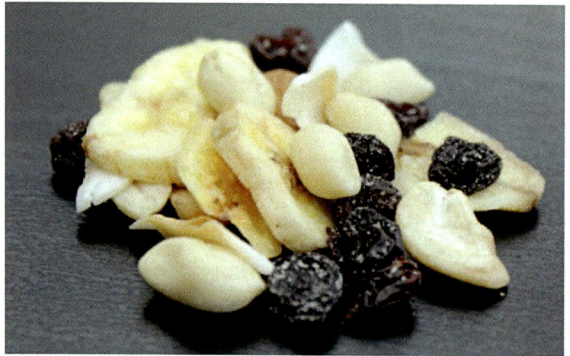

Approximately 100 calories

Sunday snack in the afternoon

Asparagus with chilli and parmesan

Ingredients

Asparagus

Chilli, garlic

Parmesan, olive oil

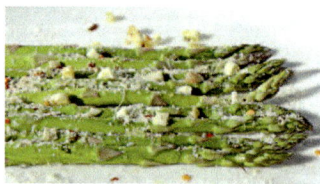

Approximately 50 calories

Sunday comes Approximately to 1250 calories

FEW RULES TO FOLLOW AND KEEP IN MIND

1) If there is something you really like for your breakfast as porridge, cereals or your favourite muesli, have it twice a week for breakfast, but for the rest, choose from clean eating breakfast.

2) If you eat a sandwich, bread, pasta, pizza, potatoes, try to have only one meal like this a day. Of course, pizza would be good just once or twice a week, no more. If you do a workout, even for 20 minutes, your body will more easily get rid of "hard to digest" calories as exercise is going to open up your veins, and the body has to pump and work harder for some time after. Otherwise, replace normal potato with sweet potato and have smaller portions of pasta.

3) Rice is the easiest to digest of the "processed carbohydrates".

4) If you are going out for dinner and you have alcohol, remember alcohol is straight carbohydrate, and your body will digest alcohol first. Try not to mix alcohol, sugar and carbs together, it's too much. Have alcohol and carb (pasta, pizza, fries, bread) if needed, but no dessert. Or have alcohol main meal (veg + protein) and dessert (no carbs), but the main meal should be meat + vegetables and have a glass with it. No guilt.

5) You can replace carb cravings for crisps, chips, and fast meals with sweet potato fries, celeriac fries, zucchini fries, turnip fries, carrot or any other root vegetables you like as fries. Chocolate cravings can be replaced with cocoa peanut butter or very rich chocolate. Then if you have a chocolate cake occasionally, it's totally fine. There is no need to be crazy.

6) If you are going to be heavily drinking in the evening, have a clean day, especially if you are losing weight, as your body is going to digest alcohol as a carb, so go clean for the morning, at lunch have smaller portions and have the dinner with alcohol.

7) If you are having a "piggy day" and you managed to stuff your face like a hamster and ate the whole peanut butter jar or had a big chocolate cake, well, I am sorry, but don't go for another lunch or dinner if you have already eaten your calories. (if someone brought a cake into the office and you had a large piece, and you feel full, cut out lunch or have lunch more as a snack).

8) If you have fast food for lunch or a late lunch, make sure your dinner is clean and a smaller portion. If dinner, make sure next day you go clean, and if you still feel full from the previous day, have smaller portions.

9) If you have alcohol in the evening with your dinner, have no processed carbs! Definitely replace them with veg or sweet potato or any clean fries or baked vegetables.

10) If you want to experience magic weight loss as celebrities do, eat clean 80% and 20% bad. Running is the fastest way to lose weight, but also do weights at least twice a week as running will make you lean and you also want to be strong.

11) Stop overcomplicating it. It's as simple as this.

12) For your stir fry up (use prawns, any meat, cheese, tofu, eggs, sea food, soya meat, garlic mushrooms).

Examples how to change your nutrition

Example 1

	MO	TU	WED	TH	FR	SAT	SUN
Break-fast	Clean ☺	Yours original	Clean	Your original	Clean	Your original	Clean
Lunch	Your Original ☹	Clean	Your original	Clean	Your original	Clean	Your original
Dinner	Your Original	Your Original	Clean	Your original	Clean	Your original	Clean
Snack	Clean	Clean	Your original	Clean	Your original	Clean	Your original
Smiley faces	☺	☹	☺	☹	☺	☹	☺
Workout	10 minutes body workout	Nothing	10min body workout	Nothing	15 minutes HIT Body	Nothing	Nothing
How you feel	Tired Good energy	Awake Sleepy					

Pay attention to how you feel the morning after your clean breakfast on Monday and how you feel on Tuesday (30 minutes AFTER the meal). If you forget, set yourself an alarm for 30 minutes and then check how your body feels. The insulin response in your body from the food you had will either make you feel tired or energetic, sleepy or awake.

You had 2 clean and 2 original meals. So, for the next week, keep a diary but add there more green than red. For at least half of the week, 3 clean and 1 original. As you wish. If you are having a bad day and you go back to your original for a day, next day make sure you go clean. But remember you are going to be a bit hungry, as your stomach will be stretched from processed carbohydrates. It will be a roller coaster for some days …

You did 3 workouts, so the following week do 4. Then add 5 minutes to each workout. So instead of 10 minutes, do 15 minutes workouts.

You want to get to 80% clean food and 20% bad. Which means 28 meals and snacks should be clean and 7 you can eat whatever you like. But after being AWARE how you feel after the healthy meals, and once your taste cells have detoxed, you might prefer the healthy choices!

There are many ways you can eat 80% clean and 20% bad. You can use ingredients which are mostly clean and add a few non-clean ingredients, but you are still winning. I will give you an example in my "normal week".

You can alternate as you like and as it suits you. But make sure you enjoy the taste of the new food, so you look forward to eating it and not just sugar or carbs.

One of the very difficult things in life is to 'break a habit'. I am giving you here 7 choices for breakfast, 7 for lunch and 7 for dinner.

For a faster and better working metabolism, the best choice for weight loss or toning up is to just focus on breakfast and dinner.

Breakfast: You will set the fast pace for your day.

Dinner: Your metabolism starts to slow down in the evening as your body knows you will soon go to sleep, and the body will rest.

If you have crazy cravings and can't resist, it is best to have 'bad food' at lunch as the body has time and chance to burn it off during the day while it's still "fast" after the breakfast (if the breakfast was clean).

If you want the best for your metabolism, then smaller portions, every 4 hours are ideal. If you have smaller portions, your body is not overwhelmed by a massive load of work, but is rather chilled and just keeps working smoothly until the evening. Just like you in the office. Lots of work involves stress. It's the same for your body.

Example 2

Some people don't have snacks.

Lets say that your most important meal is dinner. You change dinner as last.

	MO	TU	WED	TH	FR	SAT	SUN
BREAK-FAST	Clean	Clean	Clean	Clean	Clean	Clean	Clean
LUNCH	Your original	Clean	Your original	Clean	Your original	Clean	Your original
DINNER	Your original	Your original	Your original	Your original	Your original	Your original	Your original
SNACKS							
SMILEY FACES							
ACTIVITY	Run outside for distance	rest	15 min hit body workout	rest	Run try to beat your last score how far you got	Rest	Rest
FEELINGS							

Pay attention to how you feel in the evening after two clean meals, before you have your original dinner.

Next week you can alternate and one day go with a "clean dinner" and the next day "your original". But try to go from 21 meals to 17 "clean meals".

You don't have to go crazy with 21 and 7, but the cleaner you eat, the more your metabolism is speeding up.

For this week of clean eating, you are limited in the use of sauces, but in your 'normal week, feel free to use soya sauce, fish sauce, tamari sauce, wine vinegar or any other vinegar you normally use. Always try to go organic if you can.

Question about fasting: I get asked this question a lot. Yes, it is good for the body, but what many people do is try to fast for a day and then around 12 o'clock or a bit later they get hungry, and they eat. And next day they try again. And then it doesn't work, so they try again. They think it's healthy, but what they are doing is slowing down the metabolism of the body, and the body has no idea what is happening.

What you want to do is either choose one day a week or fortnight or one day a month. Then try a fast and if you feel like you are going to faint and need to eat, just eat. Write down how you felt and until what time. Next time you just try to beat it and last longer until you make it for a day. If you are going to be fasting a few times a week and not be able to make it, you will do more damage than good. Just choose a day and stick to it. The next day eat normally, and don't worry, and try again on your next set day. As a help, you can drink fruit tea with honey or maple syrup, so the sugar will help you keep going.

If you eat porridge in the morning, any breakfast bars or cereals, do not expect weight loss. If you really like it, have it 2-3 times a week and find a healthier option for the rest of the week.

When it comes to shakes and smoothies, choose any fruit or veg you like. If you like a sweet taste, use honey, maple syrup, peanut butter.

If you want to go the extra mile with clean eating, you could make homemade almond milk, coconut milk or cashew milk. I use organic full fat milk as I don't have a cow at home. If you can, use full fat milk as it's less processed than semi-skinned milk. The same with cheese. Use full fat, a hard block, not grated and where possible organic. And butter unsalted, organic, from grass fed cows. Cold pressed oils, olive oils.

If you are either endomorph, mesomorph or ectomorph, you will either get away more or less with not eating clean. You know yourself if you have problems with weight. I am lucky as I get on my own nerves the moment I put the weight on as I feel I am out of breath all the time. Lucky for me, I know very well not to mix processed sugar and carbs together very often. And when I know I am going to have processed food, I am simply good and then can enjoy a chocolate cake, as we are humans and not robots. Sometimes chocolate cake and sometimes a bottle of wine is needed to stay balanced. And yes, I am a personal trainer, and I am happy to say that. I don't want to be grumpy and cry because I just failed my diet. We only live once. Let's enjoy food. If you eat more clean, you can enjoy the chocolate cake or occasional bottle of wine without guilt, as there is no need for a crazy diet rollercoaster; there are plenty of other rollercoasters to ride!

The most stupid thing I hear from people is personal trainers would never touch chocolate. You must know yourself and remember when you were a child, the more you were told don't do this or don't go there, the temptation was irresistible. Don't do it to yourself. Learn how to control cravings, use a few tricks I've described and learn to love your body and look after it. Your only vehicle for this lifetime…….

Example 3 Emotions

	MO	TU	WED	TH	FR	SAT	SUN
BREAK-FAST	Handful peanuts	Eggs	Smoothie	Small banana	Eggs	Handful peanuts	Peanut butter sandwich
LUNCH	4 cream toffee meringues and Ritter Sport chocolate	Oven baked veg with sprinkled parmesan	Chicken salad	Butternut squash soup	Sea bass and veg	The Goodness bowl	Roast dinner with veg (no potatoes) (It's ok dish)
DINNER	Haloumi stir fry	Salmon and salad	Bag of 6 donuts	Salad with olives, tomatoes and mozarella	Pizza and bottle of wine	Curry with celeriac fries	Roasted kale, asparagus and bowl of veg from lunch Glass of wine
SNACKS	Pear	Spoonful of peanut butter Apple		Spoonful of cocoa peanut butter		Orange Banana	

I am also human, and yes, I am an emotional eater. Sometimes it's just needed. But luckily, I know how to get around it. Many people used to ask me, and I hate to lie about it. So, I am going to show you what I do when my week is an emotional rollercoaster. I will show you a "bad week', and I will explain in a simple way how I do it when things get out of control.

On *Monday,* I got told off for something by my boss, and I got angry and emotional as it was unfair, but he would not even let me finish a sentence. Never mind. I was fuming, and the first thing I did, I stopped at the shop on my way home and went crazy with sugar. I finish at 12.

Don't panic. The morning was ok, and snack was ok. I had a crazy lot of sugar during lunch time. But knowing not to mix sugar and processed carbs, and frankly I felt a bit sick after I managed to finish the chocolate as well, this is more than enough for lunch. I can't fit in anymore, anyway. But knowing it was not so good, I made sure dinner was very light and absolutely not processed carbs as the amount of sugar was high, and if I had carbs as well, my body would store the carbs as fat. I had no snack either as the amount of calories and sugar was so high my body would give me a slap if it could, so I gave it a break with a snack as I am sure it's busy enough to burn off the sugar. And I still felt a little sick from the sweetness of my lunch. Emotions ☹

On *Wednesday,* I was craving sugar badly, and I would kill for some doughnuts. This usually happens after you have had a large amount of sugar, as it's addictive, and the body creates cravings to get the dose. As I just needed donuts and I knew I will possibly eat them all in the evening, and yes, as bad as the whole bag, as I am one of those people when I open a bag of something, I usually end up eating it all. I decided to stay away from snacks and had a light lunch as the doughnuts were irresistibly tempting.

On *Thursday*, as I had (another) emotional day and I knew I overshot it with doughnuts on Wednesday, I made sure all my dishes were clean. And to make sure I will not have some crazy sugar cravings, I had a spoonful of cocoa peanut butter.

On *Friday*, I knew we were having pizza for dinner, so I had two clean meals, no snacks and then pizza and wine in the evening. I was only planning for a glass of wine, but the movie was rather good, and a bottle disappeared.

On *Sunday*, I did not have potatoes as they are harder for the digestive system to breakdown and burn (that's why we replace them mostly with sweet potato, butternut squash, celeriac fries, turnip fries or zucchini). And as I had a bit of an emotional week and fancied a glass of wine, I decided to leave snacks out. Alcohol or wine is a straight carbohydrate for your body, and it's a "poison", so your body will burn and use calories from alcohol first to get rid of them. That's why it's not great to have alcohol and another processed carb too often, as it's too much.

As a personal trainer, I would tell myself off for doughnuts and meringues, but I am also human and if there is a personal trainer that has no emotional outbursts, well, fair play to them. The magic is to eat more clean than processed, speed up the metabolism with breakfast and don't mix processed carbs and sugars together too much and too often.

Another example of how to change it:

	MO	TU	WED	TH	FR	SAT	SUN
BREAK-FAST	Clean	Original	Original	Clean	Clean	Original	Clean
LUNCH	Original	Clean	Original	Clean	Original	Clean	Original
DINNER	Clean	Original	Original	Clean	Clean	Original	Original
SNACKS							
SMILEY FACES							
ACTIVITY							
FEELINGS							

Slowly work towards more green.

My diary, as many people ask me what I eat.

	MO	TU	WED	TH	FR	SAT	SUN
BREAKFAST	Spoon of peanut butter and coffee	Smoothie	Small banana coffee	walnuts and dried papaya	Eggs	Handful of peanuts	Eggs
LUNCH	Sweet potato fries with salmon	Peanut butter sandwich with strawberries	Sushi	Broccoli cream soup	Veg salad with mustard dressing	Peanut butter stew	The goodness bowl
DINNER	Cold salad with avocado peanuts, cheese, olive oil.	Stir veg fry up with halloumi	Celeriac fries with cheese chilly balls and glass of wine	Chicken salad	Take away pizza (I have half) handful fries and about 4 onion rings	Stir fry up with sea bass Glass of wine or more	Fried veg with cheese and dressing
SNACK	Small banana	….	Peanut butter	Handful of pistachios Banana	Berries	……..	Bag of crisps

I am one of those people that really struggle to eat in the morning. I wouldn't eat until noon if I didn't have to. I just need coffee, and that's it. But I know that if I do this, my metabolism will be very slow, and I will be putting body fat on.

I have a teaspoonful of peanut butter while I have the kettle on, so I give a kick to my metabolism to get to work, and therefore, it's going to be much faster than if I ate nothing at all. I get up at 6am in the morning, so around 10 o'clock, I have a small banana or pear.

For people that don't like to eat in the morning next to your coffee maker at home, have a small bowl of nuts. If you are allergic to nuts, you could cook yourself an egg the day before and have it before you go to work. Or have a few bits of dried coconut, papaya or a small spoonful of coconut fat to get your metabolism to work. If you skip it, your body will tend to keep the fat that is coming later on and store it as fat.

If you look at my Tuesday morning, I skipped the snack as I fancied a peanut butter sandwich, and bread is very heavy for digestion. I cut out the snack to have a smaller number of calories, as I knew I was going to have an 'unhealthy' lunch.

The same on Wednesday, as I love cheese, and I knew I am going to have a bit more than I should, so I skipped the snack again.

The day after I had take-away pizza. I just ate a little less than normal, as pizza is a heavy and processed food.

If you know you are going out for dinner in the evening, eat a little less than you would normally. If you are losing weight and you are going out, choose carefully and don't mix processed carbs and sugar. You can have meat and veg if you fancy something sweet later on. If you have a dessert and you had potatoes, or fries and a glass of wine, it would be too much for your body, and you know that heavy feeling. Have either desert and veg as a side and a drink or have a meal with carbs (fries or potato) but don't have dessert. If you mix desert and processed carb + a drink, it's too much for the digestive system.

Choose and enjoy it. Next week you can alternate. If you are at home and having a glass of wine, make sure you don't have processed carbs, pasta, pizza, bread in the evening, as it's very heavy, but have veg as a side and your carbs intake. Mix it up once or twice a week if you have to. More good than bad, that's all you need to aim for. When it comes to your evening meals, if you have a sweet tooth and you really want to have a cake in the evening have a veg stir fry up and cake. But don't mix carbs with sweets. It's too much.

Don't drive yourself crazy with it. It's food, and it's meant to give you joy. Eat more clean, and you are getting there. Slowly, but surely.

In simple terms:

- Eat less pasta, pizza, bread and processed food. Use cold pressed oils, full fat or half fat and more organic.
- Avoid more processed flour and sugar.
- Find clean food you like and eat it more often.
- Eat more whole foods.
- If out: Eat clean all day and smaller portions, as the evening might be heavy food. When out eat slower as you might feel like you were missing out on something all day if you had smaller portions. Be more aware and mindful.
- Pay attention to how you feel 30 mins after meals.

For cooking as I took my week to limit and I understand people don't have the time to make their own veg stock and cook ingredients from raw. If buying canned products go organic (examples: chickpeas, coconut milk, vinegars, soya sauce, tamari sauce, lentils, beans, milk).

People ask me if I eat mayonnaise, ketchup and other sauces. Yes, I do. But as I don't eat as much processed food, I don't eat them so often.

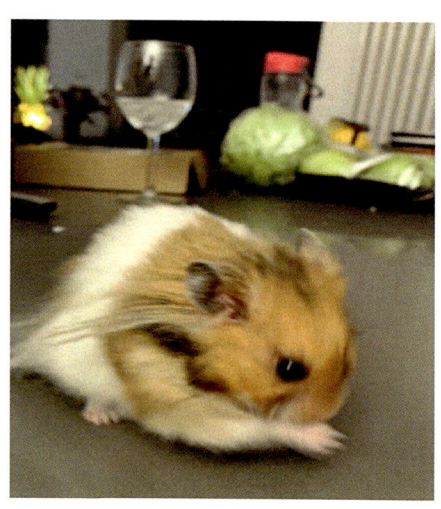

Chapter 10

THAT PLACE CALLED THE GYM & THE FACE OF CHANGE

Let's say that you hate exercise. Ok.

I am not going to persuade you here to go to the gym, even though I should, as it was my job for a long time. The benefits of exercise are great. Some people hate exercise and the gym, and it's ok. Not everyone loves it.

But I am sure you can find something that you enjoy. You don't have to do it if you don't want to, of course, but get out on a bike a few times a month, go skiing occasionally, go for a swim and have a sauna or play football with your kids in the garden. Ask your friend to join a yoga class with you and go for a drink afterwards and have some "me time". Whatever it is you like, make sure you find the time to do it.

I have good news for you. If you want to be slim, you don't really need to exercise five times a week. As I mentioned before, if you want to be slim, eat well, and if you want to be slim and look good, exercise as well. In the previous chapter, I admitted to you that I am human like you, and I do not have perfect control over food and exercise and emotions. I occasionally have a bad day, and I use sugar and the odd bottle of wine to help me cope, but I simply don't do it every day. And not every day is a bad day. But what is the difference between you and me? I know what to do when I have a crazy day and end up eating everything that I find around the house. Alcohol included.

The gym. Let's have a look at it if you struggle with it. Maybe you want to go to the gym but don't know where to start.

You may be surprised to hear that many people go to the gym because they don't want to be at home. Maybe it's a little sad. Many go there as they don't want to be at home alone, and many have this good habit as they know how exercise makes them feel. So whatever concerns you have about going to the gym, don't! You might make new friends, maybe meet the love of your life. Mentally it's going to give you the strength you need, and remember people are nice and many will be happy to help, as they also had to start somewhere.

Many have the same goal as Jolene and hope that they will be of more value to someone, feel sexier, and not think that they need to turn the light off in the bedroom in front of their partners. Many don't like their bodies and feel as if they are not good enough, as they are brainwashed like many of us, after being told what beauty is. One minute a small butt is great, and a few years later, a large size is great, so they are trying to get whatever is "in" so they fit in better. Remember the one you have got is great and it's yours. If you don't like the size of it, I will explain how to change it!

Gym and exercise

I don't have the time...

This is a classic argument from people, and sometimes I do not have the time either. It's ok.

We are all busy. Most of us are. But how much time a day do you spend on social media? Scrolling down and wasting time on what make-up is best and what new healthy product is going to help you lose weight? We all do it to some extent. My advice? And what do I do when I get busy?

I have a sister. A biological one. When I visited her for a couple of days, she started to ask me how to get rid of her belly fat. She has a fancy cross-trainer which is used as a clothes hanger as well as a swimming pool at home. In the evening, she sits on the sofa and drinks white wine spritzer and surfs the internet. I asked her, "do you have 5-10 minutes a day?". She looked at me, and I knew she was thinking it depends on what I am after. In the evening, she sits drinking her wine, and I asked her, "do you want to get a workout done in 5-10 minutes?". You don't need more than that. The answer was a raised eyebrow, and she said, "do I have to?".

So, what do I do when I am busy and have no time to go to the gym? Small steps are good....

What do I do?

Before a shower or bath, if I was really busy or was too lazy to do anything:

2 sets:

20 squats

20 mountain climbers

20 push ups or knee push ups

20 sit ups

20 shoulder overhead presses with dumb bells

It takes me roughly 5 minutes ...

Sometimes all I do is:

40 sit ups and 40 body weight squats

You will be surprised, but after a week, it's going to make a difference.

You can go on YouTube and find:

Monday: 5 – 10 minute upper body workout

Tuesday: 5 – 10 minute lower body workout

Wednesday: 5 -10 minute upper body workout

Thursday: 5 -10 minute lower body workout

Friday: 5 -10 minute HIT workout

Saturday & Sunday off.

If you want someone to guide you, my friend is doing very simple short workouts 10-15 minutes.

https://bit.ly/LenkaUrbankova

Benefits

You will get your heart rate up, which is going to speed up your metabolism for a while. You're going to feel stronger after a week, and if you feel comfortable, then next week, you will search for 10 minute workouts as you realise you do have 5 minutes a day.

We were told…. if your client keeps on telling you BUT my kids, my wife, my husband, my boss, my mother … simply do not waste your time as everyone has 20 minutes a day. I started with 5. Everyone has 5 – 10 minutes a day. There is no excuse.

Other options?

Monday / Wednesday / Friday; find yourself a 15-20 minutes HIT cardio workout to do at home if the gym is too scary or not the place you want to go to.

Or Tuesday / Thursday / Saturday; do 15-20 minutes whole body workout. Whichever one you prefer and you are going to enjoy.

You are going to feel better mentally and physically. To start with, make small changes towards clean eating. You might think this is not going to make any difference. Trust me, it will.

Just before a bath or shower is great to do short workout, as the hot water will be therapeutic and your muscles will relax after the workout. Enjoy your little siesta. There are no excuses not to do it, only the ones you create.

It is important to find something that you enjoy. As many people have a lot of stress, yoga offers stress relief, and you don't have to be fit. You will sleep well after a yoga workout. Whatever it is you are going to choose to do is up to you. All I want you to do is fall in love with a little self-care.

Whatever it is you are going to do. Gym, yoga … that craving of feeling good will be there in small doses.

How do you start?

Ok, if you want to start running, as I mentioned before, running is the fastest way to lose weight.

Why? Simply because your whole body is moving, and you are using pretty much all the muscles in your body, you have to carry your whole body weight.

Remember that every time you get a little out of breath during the day or evening, your body has to speed up. The veins open up, and blood flows faster, and your metabolism has to speed up getting nutrition and sugar to the muscles and the working organs. I can give you a massive speech on how long to run to burn body fat. Forget it!

If you run

Create a diary and in the first week, monitor how much running you do and how fast.

Next week try to beat yourself. Either on speed or distance. Only in this way are you going to get improvements. Small improvements are great, even 10 seconds faster than last week.

You might have noticed that many trainers of celebrities are achieving a "magic" weight loss. What many do is cardio in the morning and strength training in the evening or the other way around, along with clean eating. It's the only way you achieve weight loss and stay healthy.

If you have a lot of weight to lose, start with beginners' videos or exercises for overweight people. There are many, so choose the one you like, or if there is something about the person you like, go for it. If you struggle with 20 minutes a workout, record how long you managed to do it. The next day do the same and check again daily. You will slowly gain muscle and strength; every day you might add 10 seconds, and set yourself a goal to work towards it. Maybe 40 seconds … in a few days, it's going to increase! Keep track of it and pay attention to how you feel. Sometimes you're going to feel tired and not get there. Don't worry, and don't make yourself feel sick.

If you start for the first week doing crunches every night before the tv, or you get up from the sofa and do sit-ups, push ups or any kind of a workout, you will see a difference in a week. If you don't see it, you will feel it. Remember those 6 weeks I mentioned earlier.

Clients have lost 7-9kgs in two months. Did they exercise? No, just switched to 80% clean eating. It really is simple. But I want you to do something for your body too, so exercise. It's great for your mind too. And you will lose more weight and body fat if you exercise as well.

Remember, exercise is here to switch you off and relax you, not to make you more stressed. If it's stressing you out, find something different.

Benefits of workouts

Cardio: increased size of the heart muscle, increased strength of contraction, increased stroke volume, increased cardiac output, reduced resting heart rate, increased blood vessel size, decreased risk of heart disease,

BLOOD VESSELS AND BLOOD: increased blood volume and haemoglobin, reduced systolic and diastolic blood pressure,

LUNGS: increased diffusion of respiratory gases, increased functional capacity during exercise.

METABOLIC FUNCTIONS: reduced body fat, increased maximal O2 intake, decreased insulin resistance,

MUSCULAR CHANGES: increased in size and number of mitochondria, increased enzymatic function within muscle cells, increased capillarization of muscles, improved perception of muscle tone,

PSYCHOLOGICAL: and I believe these benefits are at least as important as the   physical. Improved self-mastery, increased social interaction, distraction from daily routine, decreased depression and anxiety.

EFFECTS ON BLOOD PRESSURE: very effective in reducing blood pressure over time.

BONES AND JOINTS: stronger ligaments, increased bone density, reduced loss of bone mass associated with age.

A book could be written on the benefits of exercise, but exercise is good for both the body and soul at the same time. It's your time, and you will function better if you exercise as your brain function and self-awareness and mastery will also improve. The body is your "sports car". Look after it. Remember, small doses are better than no doses at all.

The guidelines we use

CARDIOVASCULAR FITNESS: Ability of heart, lungs and muscles to take in, utilise and transport oxygen. (Running, cardio)

MUSCULAR STRENGTH: Maximum amount of force your muscle or a group of muscles can generate during a workout. Lifting heavy objects, so for example, twice a week doing squats and deadlifts, even if using smaller weights or just your body weight in case you don't like to go to the gym.

MUSCULAR ENDURANCE: Ability of muscle or groups of muscle to contract repeatedly without fatigue for a period of time. (HIT)

FLEXIBILITY: Range of movement about a joint or series of joints (yoga, great benefits for your mental well-being)

For this reason, if possible for you, it's really good to change exercises sometimes as you will be practising most of the above. Your general fitness will improve, and you will not be getting bored with repeating the same workouts.

Warm up before a workout

If you have been sitting in the office or car all day and then you jump on the treadmill full on, you can imagine how you are going to feel.

Sick, most likely.

You know what type of exercise you are going to do. If it is running, you will be using large muscle groups in your legs. Stretching your glutes and hamstrings will be beneficial, but sometimes just running at a low intensity will be enough for the first 10 minutes. You are giving your body time to slowly adjust to a workout and wake up. By stretching, you reduce the possibility of an injury as you mobilize the joints and muscles that will be used during the workout.

YouTube: 5 minutes warm up stretches for runners

Guidelines for reducing mortality and improving fitness are

3-5 times a week

60-90% of maximum heart rate (in simple terms, you need to sweat; be out of breath a little)

20-60 minutes total

You can set yourself a goal of 60 minutes a week of exercise. If you choose whole body workouts or running or any other workouts that get your heart rate high, that's all you need.

Ok, so let's say that you are unfit. It's ok. You start to work out, and for the first week, you might only end up running or on the cross trainer for 5 minutes. If you are struggling with running, the cross trainer is a great replacement, and it's not such a heavy workload for your joints. Set yourself a goal of 20 minutes. You don't have to do 20 minutes that day, but each day add a few seconds, and you will soon get there.

If you start training three times a week, even for 10 minutes, it's great. You will realize you are slowly getting better, and the next week, you will manage 12 minutes. You will slowly start to improve your cardio fitness. Exercise plus food = results!

If you think whilst running on the treadmill or on the cross trainer that you have had enough, we test it by asking the client a question. If the client can answer without too much difficulty, we know that they are not trying hard at all and in fact, it's your mental process that says I have had enough. Try to tell yourself a sentence, and if you can, I would carry on.

For many people, if they can't see any changes pretty quickly, their enthusiasm fades. If you keep a diary with your improvements in exercise and weight loss, your motivation is going to be much higher as you can see your progress. If you keep doing the same exercise and haven't made many changes when it comes to clean eating, any improvement will be small, and you will soon give up. Each week you should see an improvement in either time, intensity or number of reps. Even if the improvement is only 2 minutes faster or 2 minutes longer. You are not a hamster; you cannot go flat out as he does straight away. If you want to get further, go slowly to start with, and you will manage more than the hamster. 70% food and 30% exercise. You can do workouts daily and end up like a hamster. Running nowhere. It doesn't work without food adjustments. The number of people that look the same after three years of workouts is too large. Don't be one of them.

If the improvements in exercise are there and you are clean eating, you are on the right path. Remember, in a few weeks, it's going to stop for a week or two; don't panic.

In the first few weeks, there might not be much weight loss as to some extent, it depends on your previous diet, but you will be getting smaller in inches. Be patient, and very soon, you will see improvements in weight loss as well. Don't get hooked up on numbers, and check your BMI using the online NHS calculator.

You have got different types of muscle fibres. For this reason, if you run a lot and don't do any strength training, you will become weak in terms of lifting weights. It's not a disaster, but if you occasionally use weights or do body weight exercises, it will benefit you massively. Don't forget your overall fitness and that doing too much of one thing is never healthy. If you feel tired, have a swim and sauna. It might be a great way to improve your health, even if it's just going to be once a month. Do spend time on yourself; your mental health will benefit massively from this. If you have a family and have no time, pursue your clean eating.

10 minutes a day comes to 70 minutes a week.

20 minutes a day comes to 140 minutes a week …

Remember the benefits for your mental health as well.

Body + Mind.

FOR THE SOUL

Face of Change

What happened to Boris?

He's done a runner. I let him out of his cage as I felt sorry for him, and he managed to find himself a place under the bath in the bathroom.

What he did not realize is that he only managed to get a bigger cage but is still totally dependent on me feeding him. Isn't he like us?

Do we go from one cage to another? Maybe a bigger one or a different one, but it's still a cage? He swapped one trap for another.

I had to let him go and accept I might never catch him.

He might feel like he is free. Every time I leave food in the bathroom, and it all goes, I imagine him stuffing his face with it and struggling to squeeze through the hole, as his head with all this food is rather huge, and the hole is small. He is like us.

Sometimes we go crazy, and we stuff our faces with food or alcohol. As if this is the last time we will have food or alcohol in our lives and we overcompensate for things that are missing in our lives, maybe freedom, maybe love, maybe just being who we really are.

Sometimes he was stuffing his face so much I wondered if he believed that this is the last time he will be getting food. How do you feel when you tell yourself this is the last time I will have chocolate or something else you are planning not to eat anymore?

Does it drive you crazy?

Food, alcohol and addictions. Sometimes we stuff ourselves, as if it's some kind of protection in case things go wrong. Seeking a false sense of security. Some of us more and some less.

Chocolate, alcohol, carbs. Some people overshoot it in times of stress, it feels like these things will help us to get through the difficult times. They give us this good feeling for a short time.

Some people have perfect control over what they eat. How? Some have no control over their lives, so having control over their food gives them a 'control' feeling.

Sometimes in life we are going to have to face a storm, and for many, it's going to feel like it's going to kill them. Every storm is scary. Many pilots flying through storms don't know if they are going to make it, and many sailors have the same feeling. They are scary. What happens after the storm? Things get clear and calm. Storms are sometimes needed, they clear the air. When you are going through the storm and feel fear and wonder if you are going to make it or survive it, fear will be clouding your mind, and sometimes small things like chocolate or anything that gives us a good feeling or safe feeling, even a fake feeling, is simply needed. Feel good, feel safe. At the end of the storm, when the sky is blue again, we realize that the storm was what we needed.

Life can be a storm, and it can be a clear blue sky. It's never the same. But it's still beautiful. Some people love rain, some hate it.

This book was written for anyone who struggles dieting or who has too much stress in life. To simply explain that we are similar and we all have difficulties, and we all need help sometimes.

We all had dreams as children, and nobody ever wants to become ill. Physically or mentally. Both are just as important. Many of us were never told how to take care of our mental health, as parents were too busy with their own personal roller-coaster marriage, family issues, or overworking themselves as they were over-compensating for something they did not sort out.

We all mess up sometimes, and we all get stuck sometimes. If there were no storms, we would never appreciate clear blue skies.

Don't get stuck on a roller-coaster or in the cage of the running wheel.

If you have problems that have solutions, sort them out. Don't put everything into f…it boxes, as it's got its limitations. One day you might not be able to put anymore in, as it's going to be too full, and you will be facing a problem that will be too much to handle.

If this happens, remember there are people who were just as 'silly' as you and experienced the explosion. They had to fix it, and they will be able to point you the right way.

Some of us have had too much crazy for one lifetime, and all the 'crazy' has affected our wellbeing.

We had to change our way of thinking and perhaps accept that we lied to ourselves for a decade, as lies were more comfortable. We had to change our thinking patterns and coping mechanisms. Maybe we chose the red pill, as the lies were too much, and we would rather see the truth eventually.

Change makes us cry, laugh, sad, angry and maybe a little crazy sometimes. How do you adapt to changes? How are you going to adapt?

Go into fight mode, it's your life.

Mistakes, errors, failures are a part of our lives. Look at how many mistakes a pianist will make before he becomes a master. And when he is a master, the music is beautiful, but it has taken years of practise and error correction.

Mistakes are your mirror. They show you who you are after you made them. They show you who people around you are after you made them. Don't be afraid to fail, it's part of our lives. To fail and to get up again. Ego and pride are not as important as they tell us they are.

Life is a roller-coaster. Don't get stuck on a ride that you don't enjoy.

The fix……

You might think I had been talking a lot about mental health problems, and many people know that they tried therapy, pills, antidepressants and many more. Many read the books and know the problem. In many cases stored emotions are the biggest problem.

And I agree. If you are in this situation, I really recommend EMDR. If EMDR is not going to work for you, read the books, and you shall be able to identify your wrong patterns and coping mechanisms. Then it's going to be hard to change your own patterns and learn new ones. You will have to be self aware and realize when you get stressed you are going back to your old unhealthy coping mechanisms. It's lots of hard work.

Sometimes the darkness or traumas will create a "brain fog" when you will struggle to see the light and the way out of this. You will be slowly losing the ability to see the light, and any positivity will sound to you as if you are lying to yourself, and it will make things worse.

You just have to work out which therapy you will choose. Depression is horrible. My best friend told me once when I was at my lowest, "Depression is at your door, isn't it?". I said, "yeah, big time". She said "Say hi to her and tell her to please f..k off now, I still have life to live!". It actually worked for me.

Sometimes a little self pity is good, as you did not deserve the crap, but don't be low too long. The longer you are there, the harder it gets to get out of that place. Look at your photo as a kid and think about what you would wish for this child.

There are really good people and really nasty people. The nasty people will be your demons as they are mentally ill, and all they have is their dark soul that is draining yours out. Educate yourself from the books on how to deal with these people.

It's a game for them, and you have to play their game to survive. By educating yourself in how to play the nasty game in case you can't avoid it, you will throw these nasty individuals off. You are not here to be bullied and to be a supply for their screwed up ego. They have a problem, not you, but you will have a problem if you don't educate yourself. Once you understand the game and start standing up for yourself, it feels amazing, and it will give you the strength to find your way out.

Take care of your soul. You only have this one.

References

Dr Robin Stern.. *Gaslight Effect*. Morgan Road; 2007

Jackson MacKenzie. *Psychopath Free*. Berkley -US; 2015

Shahida Arabi. *Becoming the Narcissist's Nightmare*. SCW Archer Publishing; 2016

Kevin Dutton. *The Wisdom of Psychopaths*. FSG Adult; Reprint edition, 2013

Janet Woititz. *Adult Children of Alcoholics*. Health Communications Inc; 1983, 1990

Scott Peck. *People of the Lie*. Touchstone; 1998

Scott Peck.*The Road Less Travelled*. Touchstone; 2003

Les Carter Ph.D. *When Pleasing You is Killing Me*. BookBaby; 2018

Oliver James. *They F.... you Up*. Da Capo Lifelong Books; 2005

Dr Joe Dispenza. *Becoming Supernatural*. Hay House; 2018

George Simon. Jr. PhD. *In Sheep's Clothing*. Parkhurst Brothers Publishers Inc; 2010

David Stafford & Liz Hodgkinson. *Codependency*. Piatkus Books; 1981

Judith Orloff, MD. *The Emapths Survival Guide*. Sounds True. 2018

Bessel Van Der Kolk. *The Body Keeps the Score*. Generic; 2015

Paul T.Mason, Ms Randi Kreger. *Stop walking on eggshells*. New Harbinger Publications;2020

Eric Berne. *Games People Play*. Dell Publishing; 1967

Laura Charanza. *Ugly Love*. BookBaby; 2018

Ernest Hemingway. *A Moveable Feast*. Scribner; Reprint edition; 2010

Martha Stout. *The Sociopath Next Door*. Broadway Books; 2005

Jane McGregor and Tim McGregor. *The Empathy Trap*. Sheldon Press; 2019

Premier Training International. *Certificate in Gym Instruction, Personal Trainer*. 2012

Websites

Mayoclinic.org

Acknowledgments

To Rashmi Loku Moolya who provided inspiration and support; I could not have done it without her.

Ken Bickers for working with me to pull the book together.

Mudr Helena Machova, psychiatrist, for support and advice.

Front cover design and cartoon by Simon Ellinas, www.caricatures.org.uk

To my many clients for inspiration and laughs along the way …

Casper (aka Boris) the hamster …

Eva Kicmerova, author and photographer …

A Covid lockdown project that has been completed!